Object matters

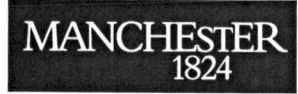

Manchester University Press

Object matters
Condoms, adolescence and time

Nicole Vitellone

Manchester University Press
Manchester and New York
distributed exclusively in the USA by Palgrave

Copyright © Nicole Vitellone 2008

The right of Nicole Vitellone to be identified as the author of this work has been asserted by her in accordance with the Copyright, Designs and Patents Act 1988.

Published by Manchester University Press
Oxford Road, Manchester M13 9NR, UK
and Room 400, 175 Fifth Avenue, New York, NY 10010, USA
www.manchesteruniversitypress.co.uk

Distributed in the United States exclusively by
Palgrave Macmillan, 175 Fifth Avenue,
New York, NY 10010, USA

Distributed in Canada exclusively by
UBC Press, University of British Columbia, 2029 West Mall,
Vancouver, BC, Canada V6T 1Z2

British Library Cataloguing-in-Publication Data is available

Library of Congress Cataloging-in-Publication Data is available

ISBN 978 0 7190 8933 6 paperback

First published by Manchester University Press in hardback 2008

This paperback edition first published 2013

The publisher has no responsibility for the persistence or accuracy of URLs for any external or third-party internet websites referred to in this book, and does not guarantee that any content on such websites is, or will remain, accurate or appropriate.

Printed by Lightning Source

Contents

	Acknowledgements	*page* vii
1	AIDS, the condom and the history of heterosexuality: an introduction	1
2	Sex education and the condom	13
3	Condoms and sex research	36
4	Safer sex representations	56
5	AIDS, pornography and the condom	78
6	The condom, gender and sexual difference	96
7	Condoms and consent	118
8	Conclusion: condoms, adolescence and time	136
	References	140
	Index	157

Acknowledgements

This book has been a long time in the making. I am grateful to Lisa Adkins who read drafts of earlier chapters and provided critical feedback. I especially want to thank Jane Kilby, Liz Wilson and Steven Angelides for their comments and suggestions on the final drafts. Their encouragement and friendship has been a source of inspiration, particularly towards the end when it mattered most. Former colleagues in MIPC at Manchester Metropolitan University taught me many good things. I also want to thank my new colleagues in the School of Sociology and Social Policy at Liverpool University for providing a supportive space in which to complete the book. The editors and reviewers at Manchester University Press gave the book a new direction. Becky Johansson kept me on track. My mates John Hobbs, Stuart Baron, Marco Ambrosio, Katy Endean, Shirley Tate, Debs Gatenby, Ash Knowles, Antonella Magnavacca, Nigel Carleton, Eleanor Casella, Helen Keane, Kirsten Farrell, Lyndall Kennedy, Marsha Rosengarten, Joanna Hodge and Linnell Secomb the biggest thank you. Finally, I want to thank my parents Antonietta and Vince and my sister Marianne for their love and support over the years.

Versions of some chapters have been published previously. Sections of chapter 4 first appeared in '"I think it more of a white person's sort of awareness": condoms and the making of a white nation in media representations of safer sex', *Feminist Media* 2002 vol. 2, no. 1, pp. 19–36. A revised version is reprinted here with the permission of Routledge. Chapter 6 first appeared as 'Condoms and the making of sexual difference in AIDS heterosexual culture', *Body & Society* 2002 vol. 8, no. 3, pp. 71–94. A revised version is reprinted here with the permission of Sage.

1
AIDS, the condom and the history of heterosexuality: an introduction

Before her death in 1990 Linda Singer made a number of observations regarding the nature of power, control and regulation in relation to sexuality. Comparing the social context of the 1980s with the 1960s she noted specific changes in the history of sexuality. This includes a shift from sexual revolution and a 'politics of ecstasy' to sexual epidemic and a 'recessionary erotic economy' (1993: 116). For Singer the former can be characterised by 'a revolutionary transformation of sexual theory, practice, and politics that would make sex better, or make better sex' (1993: 113). These transformations included a depriviliging of 'heterosexism over homosexuality and lesbian experience, phallocentricty over gynocentricity, reproductive over non-reproductive sex' (1993: 115). But with the rise of the sexual epidemic of AIDS 'an ecstatic carnival is progressively being displaced by a more sober and reserved aesthetic of "sexual prudence and body management". The language of "better sex" is being replaced by that of "safe sex" and the promotion of a "new sobriety"' (Singer, 1993: 116). Whilst Singer observed that these changes have been most apparent in relation to gay men's lives she hypothesised that issues of body management would eventually have an impact on other social groups and would persist for some time. Singer also pointed out, following Foucault, that the sexual epidemic of AIDS 'provides an occasion and a rationale for multiplying points of intervention into the lives of bodies and populations' (1993: 117). She therefore warned that the current age of sexual epidemic requires a new sexual politics and a 'rethinking of the relationship between bodies, pleasures and powers beyond the call for liberation or repression' (1993: 116–117). Written almost twenty years later, this book carries on Singer's less than optimistic view of safer sex discourse and considers the relationship between bodies, pleasures and power in the current organisation of sexuality. It does so in relation to the object of the condom. It is the presumption of this book that the discourse of safer sex initiates specific modes of regulation which concern the condom itself.

In a critical discussion of the contemporary meaning of the condom Joshua Gamson makes a series of claims which are later called into question by Scott Bravmann. This debate was published in *The Journal of the History of Sexuality* (1990, 1991). The 'Rubber Wars' were primarily concerned with mapping the shifting meaning of the condom and in particular its significance in the late twentieth century. For Gamson, the initiator of the debate, the popular meanings of the condom post-1980s include: 'a sign of sexual license, a sign of sexual maturity, a sign of AIDS awareness, a cumbersome piece of rubber and so on' (1990: 263). What interests Gamson are the battles over the condom's meaning. In particular, he is interested in how the condom comes to mean certain things at certain times, and how it comes to be associated with certain behaviours and uses whilst being disassociated from others. Indeed he argues 'it is given a power afforded few inanimate objects' (1990: 263).

In addressing historical aspects of the condom in the US Gamson asks the following questions: 'How do objects become endowed with meaning? How do meanings shift? What conditions underlie and affect the construction of these meanings? What difference does an object's uses – for example, a sexual use – make for this process?' (1990: 263). Despite these broad-ranging questions, Gamson provides some straightforward answers. The condom, he argues, has two possible meanings. First, a contraceptive-prophylactic meaning and, second, a sexual one with connotations of sexual intercourse (1990: 266). But it is the question of *who* is constructing the meaning of the condom that interests Gamson the most. Comparing the 1940s with the 1980s he suggests that the main actors in the battle over its meaning have changed somewhat. Whilst manufacturers continue to shape the object's meaning, Gamson points out that the US battles over the condom during the 1940s took place in the courtroom and concerned issues of availability and distribution; in the 1980s the site of meaning shifts from the courts to the media, that is 'from legality to publicity' (1990: 280). In addressing the impact of the media and advertising in transforming the condom's meaning in the 1980s, Gamson argues, 'the condom has now been marketed as not-a-contraceptive: it is a beauty aid, a personal hygiene item, a public service – all, however euphemistically, based on the prevention-of-disease frame and a desexualization of the condom' (1990: 274).

Although Gamson stresses the importance of addressing the framing aspects in giving the 'condom a makeover, from sleazy to "smart"' (1990: 273), he concludes that focusing on advertising and media practices alone is somewhat limited in providing a social history of the condom in the context of AIDS. Such an approach, he argues, does not address either the reception of safer sex media messages or indeed the relationship between the public's interpretation of 'what the condom is and their use of the object' (1990: 281). According to Gamson, people's definitions are affected by cultural understandings which 'differ across social groupings (race, class, gender, age) as well as across time' (1990: 281). This point and other elements of Gamson's account of the 'Rubber Wars' are critically addressed in Scott Bravmann's response. Bravmann's main criticism concerns the omission of sexuality from Gamson's 'list of "social grouping" that inform individuals' understandings of condoms' (1991: 101). The problem with this omission, argues Bravmann, is twofold. By deleting sexuality from a list of social groupings Gamson erases a particular social history of the condom in the context of AIDS. More specifically, Gamson erases the sexualisation of the condom by gay men and lesbians via the eroticisation of safer sex and the deployment of condoms for the purpose of covering 'penises, dildoes, boots, and so on; when cut open lengthwise, they work well as dental dams for use during oral-anal and oral-vaginal contact' (Bravmann, 1991: 99). It is these particular uses and understandings of the condom by queer sexualities which Gamson's sociological account is considered to deny. As Bravmann puts it, 'Gamson effectively denies that lesbians and gay men possess any significant power or knowledge – not even enough to distinguish our own cultural understandings of the condom from those of heterosexual women and men' (1991: 101).

And this leads to Bravmann's critical observation about Gamson's account of the meaning of the condom – its latent heterosexism. More specifically, Bravmann argues that the omission of the adjective heterosexual before the terms sex or sexual intercourse assumes and takes for granted that all sex is the same, that is, heterosexual intercourse. The problem is compounded by Gamson's definition of the contraceptive-prophylactic meaning of condom use. 'In short, his approach obliterates queer sexualities by failing to clarify that in lesbian and gay male sexual practices condoms have no "double function"' (Bravmann, 1991: 99). That is, by claiming that the condom is used as *both* a disease prevention device and a form of birth control Gamson is understood to privilege its role in heterosexual intercourse and thus re-essentialise the object, even though, as Bravmann points out, Gamson wants to avoid fixing the meaning of the condom. Bravmann thus concludes: 'lesbians and gay men are scarcely visible in his picture' (1991: 102).

In his response to Bravmann, Gamson (1991) welcomes the extension of the 'Rubber Wars' to theoretical analysis. Gamson then proceeds by qualifying his points. First, he qualifies his use of the term discourse to 'hegemonic discourse' and makes it clear that his analysis concerns public debates around the condom and the *dominant* discourse of safer sex in advertising and the mass media. In other words, Gamson suggests that, far from excluding sexuality in his history of the condom and thus erasing gays and lesbians from the picture, his analysis serves to demonstrate how meaning is created by certain actors in certain contexts within dominant discourse. In his reply Gamson reiterates 'whatever one's assessment, let us be clear: to believe that a group of people is marginalized in a discourse, and therefore to treat them as marginal in an analysis of that discourse, is not to advocate or reinforce the marginalization of those people' (1991: 103). And this leads to his second point of qualification. Gamson stresses the limitations of simply focusing on the framing elements of the condom in advertising and the mass media and reiterates the necessity of looking to private definitions for understandings of how meanings are created. 'Bringing in a study of gay and lesbian sexual practices surrounding condoms could then be tremendously revealing academically (as well as of interest in its own right): it might shed light on how and why certain people are able to ignore or resist meanings that are asserted as absolute but enacted in struggles that essentially exclude them' (Gamson, 1991: 104).

Within this response Gamson makes a series of moves that warrant further consideration. Whilst the study of gay and lesbian sexual practices would indeed be revealing academically, especially in relation to questions of interpretation and resistance to dominant safer (hetero)sex discourse, sexual knowledge is not confined to advertising and the mass media. Sexual knowledge in any historical moment and national context, as Porter and Hall (1995) point out, is gathered from a range of sources. From the mid-twentieth century this includes information gathered from sex education in schools, the publication of sex surveys and public debates such as feminist debates on pornography as well as bodily responses and social practices. In this book I investigate sexual knowledge in the era of AIDS from within these sites. Focusing on the period 1986 to 1996 I examine the significance of the condom in the school classroom (Chapter 2), mass-media public health campaigns (Chapter 4), feminist debates on pornography (Chapter 5) and sex research on adolescent sexual practices (Chapter 3) as well as young people's experiences of the condom in the sexual encounter (Chapters 6 and 7). My analysis throughout the book examines the history of AIDS in relation to sexual knowledge about the condom. In so doing this book addresses the changing meaning of the condom in the mid-1980s from a contraceptive device to a barrier against HIV. Focusing on the British, Australian and US governments' response to the threat of a heterosexual AIDS epidemic, *Object Matters* considers the impact of three somewhat different approaches to HIV/AIDS education. In particular, this book examines the constituent effects of comprehensive, abstinent only and restricted sex education policies for the regulation of western adolescent sexuality. Whilst others have focused on the denial of youth sexuality in AIDS education messages, particularly in sub-Saharan Africa, and the impact of such denial in increasing HIV rates amongst youth (see Campbell, 2003; Campbell, Nair and Maimane, 2006), this book takes a different approach. By focusing on three western social contexts in which AIDS education has been targeted at youth, my aim is to address the consequences of sex education messages about condom use for adolescent sexuality.

The omission of sexuality in Gamson's account of the condom is unfortunate. Nonetheless it is significant to note that Gamson – and Bravmann to some degree – finds that sexuality, along with race, class and gender, *impacts* on the condom's meaning. That is, social groupings precede the definition of the condom. The meaning of the condom in these accounts is thus understood to be socially determined. In this sense there appears to be little consideration of how gender, race, class *and* sexuality may be constituted in particular ways by the discourse of safer sex. My argument in this book is that such social divisions and social identities are formed precisely in relation to the condom and more specifically in relation to the practices of safer (hetero)sex and the consumption and reception of safer sex messages. Instead of thinking of sexuality as outside of this process, my analysis of what the condom is and does in the post-AIDS period shows how the condom constitutes sexuality in particular ways.

Both Simon Watney's analysis of the British media and Leo Bersani's account of the US press in the 1980s critically address the construction of sexuality in AIDS representations. Commenting in the first decade of the epidemic, Watney finds that the media communications industry presents AIDS as a property of particular groups, specifically gay men. Moreover, he suggests that even when the dominant discourse of AIDS in the media presented the virus as one which also affects the heterosexual population, gay men were still blamed for the transmission of HIV. What troubles Watney is not just the content of these media discourses but theoretical analyses of such representations by cultural commentators. In particular, Watney has serious reservations about the effectiveness of a plague analogy and moral panic theory to address the history of AIDS representations.

The strengths of moral panic theory, as Watney points out, lay with its ability to identify the role of the media in constructing a discrete social problem. In the context of AIDS, the perceived threat posed by certain groups in the early 1980s, particularly gay men, is identified as an effect of media representations which label sexual behaviours and individuals as both the source and cause of concern. Although such a move ultimately disentangles the notion of deviance from 'homosexuality', and foregrounds the social context in which the homosexual and homosexuality are labelled as such, the costs of the moral panic theory according to Watney far exceed its benefits. In prioritising the social processes through which certain groups are labelled as other, and gay men in particular have been labelled as monsters, deviants and guilty victims, this analysis simply reiterates the marginalisation of gays and lesbians in relation to dominant AIDS discourse and does not therefore recognise gay men as a social group. Such an approach 'serves to further regulate and reinforce the workings of modern sexual categories by seemingly forcing together all the varieties of homosexual desire and identity into a monolithic totality, faced by an equally monolithic heterosexuality' (Watney, 1994: 13). The danger here is that moral panic theory both 'avoids the whole question of how desire operates to motivate particular sexual behaviours' (Watney, 1994: 13) and at the same time fails to address the more important issue of how AIDS has been mobilised to constitute not so much the Other but, rather, the normative. Watney's analysis both highlights the problem of thinking about AIDS simply in relation to the Other and suggests that AIDS representations concern the regulation of (hetero)sexuality. It is this issue which this book aims to address.

A further point of contention for Watney concerns the technical application of moral panic theory to the historical moment of AIDS. As he points out, the definition of a moral panic is a sudden, distinct event that spontaneously appears and then disappears once the necessary government interventions have been made to deal with the 'problem'. And yet, as Watney argues, 'AIDS' has not simply disappeared but has rather remained a constant panic. Moreover, he suggests that the nature of this panic concerns the regulation of sexuality, especially in matters concerning public representations (Watney, 1994: 8). According to Watney, persistent media reports of children's sexuality, together with the ongoing debates about sex education in schools and public representations of sex, 'all orchestrate the larger question of sexuality itself, as if it were something intrinsically dangerous' (Watney, 1994: 9). Taking up Watney's concerns, this book shows how western media reports and debates about the condom in the 1980s and early 1990s involved not so much issues of danger but the production and regulation of adolescent (hetero)sexuality.

Watney's work also draws attention to the way AIDS representations have been analysed in relation to previous histories of sexually transmitted diseases. Historians and critics have observed the use of plague imagery in representations of HIV/AIDS and shown how such imagery is problematic (Brandt, 1987; Gilman, 1988; Mort, 2000). Whilst such historical accounts have been useful in illustrating the rhetoric around AIDS, especially during the initial period of the epidemic, Watney (1994) argues that locating AIDS within the history of contagious diseases displaces a consideration of 'the irreducible specificities of HIV and its multiple collisions with the late twentieth century' (1994: 272). Watney's greatest concern is that the metaphor of plague 'naturalises the impact of HIV amongst gay men, and displaces attention away from the direct consequences of homophobic denial of Safer Sex education to those in the greatest need – a denial which may be accurately tallied in our mounting mortality statistics' (Watney, 1994: 276).

Not much appears to have changed since the mid-1980s. In 2005 the British government was still reluctant to acknowledge the reality of the HIV epidemic as one which continues to affect predominantly gay men and increasingly Black Africans living in Britain. In its efforts to educate the general public about HIV the government presented the virus as a threat to white heterosexuals even though 'gay men are 90 times more likely to be positive' (Scott-Clark and Levy, 2005: 30) and account for 43 per cent of those with HIV and yet they constitute only 1 per cent of the population (Scott-Clark and Levy, 2005: 26). The £50 million AIDS campaign featured posters of celebrities photographed with their hands clasped over their ears or mouths. Below the photograph the words 'Hear no evil, See no evil, Speak no evil' appear in bold. 'The message is clear: when it comes to sex and HIV, we are not listening' (Scott-Clark and Levy, 2005: 26). Scott-Clark and Levy (2005: 26) raise the obvious question: what has led the government to commit millions to such a health campaign when very few white British heterosexual men and women have contracted HIV in the UK? 'If the government's aim in concealing the true story of HIV has been to protect sections of the British society from stigma, what a dreadful mess it has made of it' (Scott-Clark and Levy, 2005: 28). In failing to specifically address those most at risk, recent national safer sex education campaigns could thus be understood to inadvertently reproduce the homophobia discussed by Watney in the 1980s.

But is this the case? Do misguided safer sex campaigns have a negative impact on gay men's sexual health? Is a young gay man's (perceived) lack of knowledge about condom use simply an outcome of homophobic AIDS education policies which marginalise particular social groups? Does this history of AIDS in Britain expose a history of homophobia? Whilst Watney, Scott-Clark and Levy appear to suggest that this is the case, Tim Dean warns against such hasty conclusions.

From 1996 the availability of HIV treatments such as triple combination therapy along with antibody testing significantly changed the meaning of HIV and safer sex amongst gay men. Whilst these new methods of assessing and managing HIV and risk *within* the body (Flowers, 2001) appear to have resulted in an increase in the prevalence of 'barebacking' (unprotected anal sex) amongst gay men, Dean (2000: 142) argues that to assume that non-use of condoms is a result of homophobia and ignorance rather than choice provides a very limited picture of social relations. In particular, Dean is critical of accounts that attribute blame to the mainstream media and the British and US governments amongst others for the rise in unsafe sex amongst gay men:

> While it was crucial in the eighties to emphasize how social forces such as homophobia and racism exacerbated the epidemic, it is foolhardy now to maintain that prejudice represents the principal impediment to effective AIDS prevention. Yet this assumption continues to pervade virtually all progressive discourse on safe-sex education, generating the fantasy that once we fine-tune educational techniques to take exhaustive account of the multiple demographic variables involved, then – together with adequate funding and thorough dissemination of this finely calibrated educational material – the safe sex message will take hold and the epidemic can be eradicated. (2000: 143)

As Dean sees it the practice of unsafe sex warrants further consideration for a number of reasons. Unsafe sex has less to do with a lack of knowledge than a passion for ignorance. Sex without a condom and the consequences it brings such as sero-conversion eliminate a level of uncertainty and anxiety from one's life by reducing the *potential* threat of HIV (2000: 152). Unsafe sex is not simply about individual decision-making, it is a social activity (2000: 140). Unsafe sex is desired not because of its physical attributes but because it holds subjective meanings for the self and for the other, meanings which concern an interdependent relationality within the sexual encounter itself (2000: 166). But how might we understand the sociality of condom *use*? And how are we to address government-funded AIDS education campaigns which promote safer sex to white *heterosexuals*? What can be said of the media discourse on condom use for the general heterosexual population? How are we to comprehend the promotion of safer sex to western heterosexuals over the past twenty years particularly when this social group has remained at low risk from HIV? These are some of the questions this book aims to address.

Following on from Watney's historical account of AIDS in the 1980s as involving a crisis of representation, and a crisis over the framing of knowledge about sexuality, Bersani (1993: 198) noted a similar disregard in the US for gay men's health and for those suffering from AIDS. Discussing the Reagan government's systematic neglect for AIDS during the 1980s, he explains the problem succinctly: 'the tendency to think of AIDS as an epidemic of *the future*, rather than a catastrophe of the present' (1993: 199, my emphasis). What stands out in Bersani's account of AIDS as an epidemic concerned with the future – as opposed to the present – is the discourse of condom use aimed at the general white heterosexual population, a social group at minimal risk:

> Try keeping up with AIDS research through TV and the press, and you'll remain fairly ignorant. You will, however, learn a great deal from the tube and from your daily newspapers about heterosexual anxieties. Instead of giving us sharp investigative reporting – on say *60 Minutes* – on research inefficiently divided among various uncoordinated and frequently competing private and public centres and agencies, or on the interests of pharmaceutical companies in helping to make available (or helping to keep unavailable) new antiviral treatments and in furthering or delaying the development of a vaccine, TV treats us to nauseating processions of yuppie women announcing to the world that they will no longer put out for their yuppie boyfriends unless these boyfriends agree to use a condom. Thus hundreds and thousands of gay men and IV drug users, who have reason to think they may be infected with HIV, or who know that they are (and who therefore live in daily terror that one of the familiar symptoms show up); or who are already suffering from an AIDS-related illness, or who are dying from one of these illnesses, are asked to sympathize with all those yuppettes agonizing over whether they're going to risk losing a good fuck by taking that 'unfeminine' initiative of interrupting the invading male in order to insist that he practice safe sex. (1993: 202–203)

From this account we could thus infer that the discourse of safer sex is one which normalised heterosex by making other sex marginal. In addition, we could surmise that the discourse of safer sex produced the truth of the condom as both interrupting male sexual pleasure and threatening women's feminine gender identity. From this account we could therefore deduce that the framing of sexual knowledge about the condom in media representations of AIDS from the mid-1980s to the mid-1990s concerns a *history of heterosexuality*.

Whilst Bersani clearly has disdain for such media representations, especially since they exclude gay men, this book takes a different approach. Throughout the book I am interested in the discourse of safer sex targeted at the general heterosexual population. In the chapters that follow I consider the history of the condom in relation to the national mass-media public health campaigns, eroticised representations of safer sex, AIDS-related sex research and school-based sex education policies as well as adolescent safer sexual practices. The approach taken in this book involves a close reading of texts and a secondary analysis of empirical research on western adolescent safer sex practices. The theorists, critics and social researchers who appear throughout the book form a body of literature concerned with the social and cultural impact of AIDS during a particular historical period of the epidemic, one which involves the threat of a western heterosexual HIV epidemic. In addressing this body of literature, especially in relation to the mainstreaming of the discourse of safer sex, I illustrate how the condom concerns a history of heterosexuality.

In Chapters 2 and 3 I consider Bersani's observation that AIDS is an epidemic of the future. Via an analysis of sex research methods and sex education policies I show how adolescent sexuality is constructed as future-oriented. In my discussion of sex education policies I also show how talk of condoms in the classroom or the banning of such talk concerns the regulation of an adolescent's future sexuality. My argument in this book is that the condom is constitutive of adolescence as a future-oriented (hetero)sexual identity. I demonstrate that an unfinished, yet-to-be complete adolescent (hetero)sexuality is uneven: it creates class distinctions and racialised divisions.

In Chapter 4 and 5 I examine the impact of representations of safer (hetero)sex from the mid- to late 1980s. Focusing on the promotion of the condom in US, British and Australian magazine advertisements, national television campaigns and pornography I consider how the condom is represented, and the ways in which safer sex representations have been researched and analysed. My analysis is concerned with practices of consumption and their social effects. In particular, I consider the relationship between representations of safer sex and processes of identity formation including gender identity, sexual identity, national identity and sexual citizenship.

In Chapters 6 and 7 I consider the materiality of the condom. My focus is young people's accounts of the condom in the sexual encounter. In these chapters I examine empirical analyses of safer sex practice which claim that the condom challenges the construction of male sexuality, threatens the performance of a masculine identity and interferes with a sexed male body-image. Taking on board these claims I ask the following questions. What does the condom do? Can we simply assume that heterosexual men don't wear condoms? Do they really interrupt male sexual pleasure? Does the condom threaten the gendered construction of male sexuality as an instinctual, spontaneous force? Is it the case that women struggle to initiate condom use with men? Do men resist safer sex? And what impact does the condom have in the communication of consent? How are we to address the issue of consent in relation to the discourse of safer sex? In addressing these questions I consider the role sex researchers and social theorists have played in producing sexual knowledge on safer sex. In answering these questions this book evaluates the object of the condom. In so doing it aims to develop a social history of the condom in the context of AIDS.

2
Sex education and the condom

This chapter analyses the social effects of sex education for adolescents. Focusing on the period post-1986, the chapter examines the impact of AIDS education, and in particular safer sex education in the classroom. The main point of concern is the framing of sexual knowledge of the condom in public secondary high schools. By comparing and contrasting the provision of sex education in the US, UK and Australia the chapter draws attention to the differences and similarities in present and past histories of sex education. In so doing the chapter seeks to highlight how the regulation of adolescent sexuality in the era of AIDS concerns the object of the condom. The overall argument is that sex education concerns the regulation of the adolescent's sexual future.

A history of sex education

Adolescence is generally understood as a transitional social category. In the early writings of Hall (1904), the experience of schooling is identified as a key process which produces the modern adolescent subject. Since schooling physically separates children from adults, whilst simultaneously prolonging the temporality of childhood, schooling and especially secondary education are understood to be constitutive of an extended transitional adolescent phase. Addressing Hall's early account of adolescence and education, Moran (2000) suggests that the modern concept of adolescence would not have emerged without the demand for sexual self-control and chastity before marriage. The passage from adolescence into adulthood was viewed by Hall as especially problematic for adolescent boys. Premature sexual development was understood to lead to degeneracy. Sexual self-control was considered necessary for the progress of Anglo-Saxon civilisation, particularly towards the end of the nineteenth century with new immigrants arriving from eastern and southern Europe. In Hall's work 'adolescent chastity not only signified the social distance between "civilized" and "primitive" races, it created this distance through a complex biological process known as recapitulation' (Moran, 2000: 16). The chaste white middle-class adolescent became demarcated from the 'savage' youth who 'was considered fully mature, sexually active, at an age when the "civilized" adolescent was just beginning his most strenuous period of mental and spiritual growth' (Moran, 2000: 17). What I want to draw out here is the idea that the white Anglo-Saxon youth becomes adolescent whereas the sexually mature and active youth goes straight from childhood into adulthood. Having defined adolescence in relation to sexual morality and racial fears, adolescent bodies now required careful and external control, a role which sex education came to play.

The provision of sex education in public schools during the first part of the twentieth century was not without controversy. The historian of sexuality Julian Carter (2001) draws attention to the conflicting views of sexual knowledge for adolescents in the US during the period 1910–40. Access to sexual information was understood to protect the nation, especially the future of the nation and the future of the American family. At the same time sexual knowledge was viewed as socially dangerous as it was presumed to 'transform itself into sexual activity' (Carter, 2001: 216). This contradiction is played out in the amount of attention given to knowledge of contagion. Instead of teaching adolescents about infection and its prevention, sex educators produced a fear of contagion. And yet knowledge of contagion was also considered dangerous as it potentially alienated women from men and thus undermined heterosexual romance, the institution of marriage and the family. Carter illustrates the problem of contagious knowledge in the sex education manuals of Irving Steinhardt. In the manual *Ten Sex Talks to Girls* (1913) there is very little information about sex. Instead girls are confronted with ghastly photographic images of a syphilitic baby which are aimed at producing sympathy for the suffering infant. According to Carter (2001: 230) the photograph and accompanying text 'Poor little syphilitic baby! No one loves you nor wants to hug and kiss you except, perhaps, the poor mother who had the misfortune of bringing you into the world' were intended to scare adolescents into chastity as well as to develop their maternal urges to cherish and care for children. 'Purity in the service of the coming generation was morally and socially superior to purity only out of fear' (Carter, 2001: 230). Such fearful sexual knowledge was contested on the grounds that the syphilitic baby was in fact a threat to the future of the family as it presented adolescent girls with a fear of men and heterosexual sex. By the mid-1920s the emphasis on prenatal contagious knowledge in sex education was replaced with developmental sex education which emphasised '"the moral, the normal, the healthy, the helpful, and the aesthetic aspects" of sex' (Carter, 2001: 233). Whilst developmental sex education presented sex as positive and natural, the aims were nonetheless similar to contagious knowledge, to restrain vice and produce virtue in adolescents.

The regulation of adolescent sexual behaviour in the early twentieth century is further illustrated in Bashford's (2004) historical account of the emergence of Australian public health. According to Bashford 'national hygiene *became* the responsibility of individual citizens' (Bashford, 2004: 173). One's own intimate sexual choices and actions were understood to be significant for the nation or race. The focus on sex hygiene constituted an extreme form of nationalism 'based squarely on the idea of white Australia: it was explicitly a nationalism of race. The pursuit ... of health, hygiene and cleanliness was one significant way in which the whiteness of white Australia was imagined' (Bashford, 2004: 3). What stands out in Bashford's account of sexual health in the Australian nation is the prominence she accords to 'eugenics itself as a kind of preventative health' (2004: 180). Bashford carefully illustrates her argument in relation to an interwar poster campaign 'Sow the Seeds of Good Health' produced by the New South Wales Department of Health in 1930. In her discussion of the accompanying text 'Through Sunshine, Fresh Air and Cleanliness' and the hyper-masculine image that exhorts women and especially men to 'take responsibility for themselves as reproductive, and therefore raced and national, beings' (2004: 178), Bashford points out that this sex education message with its emphasis on sex as a reproductive and potentially dangerous act is geared towards the governance of individuals' sexual health not so much for their own sake as for the sake of the next generation. 'Eugenic culture and its public health expressions problematised the sexual and racial connection between the present generation and its progeny – one, two, one hundred generations into the future' (2004: 166). What I want to take away from Bashford's analysis is the point that eugenic public health connects the reproductive (hetero)sexual citizen to a *future*-oriented project, one whereby the concern is to protect the health of unborn *future* generations and in so doing the whiteness of white Australia.

How might this understanding of public health as concerning a *future*-oriented project inform a history of safer sex education for adolescents? Is it useful to read the history of sex education in the context of AIDS in relation to a previous historical past? Or does such an analysis obscure an understanding of the history of the condom post the mid-1980s? To think about how it might be possible to invent a different history of the present I begin by sketching out the provision of sex education from the postwar period.

In his book *Dangerous Sexualities* the social historian Frank Mort (2000) makes a series of connections between the past and the present history of British sex education and argues for a 'need to construct modes of history-writing which grasp that *past/present* relation' (2000: 165, my emphasis). In Mort's account public reactions to AIDS connect with early nineteenth-century beliefs about health and disease as they concern ideas of moral and immoral sex and dangerous sexualities. Using the example of a newspaper article from 1983 which associates San Francisco's homosexual community with AIDS, Mort argues that such accounts are 'framed by moral condemnation, reaffirming the distance between our own sexuality and "deviant" pleasures' (2000: 166). By the late 1980s, and with the realisation that the entire heterosexual population is at risk, 'the moral *frisson* ... shifted register. No longer is it generated by fascination with deviance – that other sexuality. Danger is everywhere' (2000: 167). The threat of AIDS to the general population propelled the British government to raise public awareness of HIV in the mass media (see Chapter 4).

The entanglement of social medicine with moral regulation in Mort's account of AIDS has its roots in the late nineteenth- and early twentieth-century English social hygiene movement. The hygiene movement, which gained momentum in the early part of the twentieth century, produced a 'renewed moral emphasis within preventative medicine' (Mort, 2000: 137) particularly in relation to the bodies of adolescents. Within this scientific discourse Mort notes the significance of 'moral pronouncements about society's *future* progress or decline' (2000: 138, my emphasis). Sex education in this context is key in 'channelling the sexual instinct towards socially approved goals' (2000: 137) and warning the public of the 'moral consequences for those who broke the laws of health' (2000: 139). Hygienists saw sex, especially for young men, as a biological instinct which 'needed to be fought, tamed and finally conquered in the progress towards physiological maturity' (2000: 152). The passage into maturity came to define white manhood with boys 'warned that only "among primitive men" were physical pleasures experienced as animal lusts' (2000: 154). The biological model of adolescent male sexuality contrasts with the earlier views of the social purists. Between the 1890s and 1920s sex education material published by purity organisations warned boys against 'the dangers of sexual sin' (Hall, 1991: 29), with masturbation considered 'the paramount sin' 'leading to fornication, disease and death, by eroding self-discipline and self-control' (Hall, 1991: 32).

The concern with boys' sexuality is also evident in the Australian context. During the 1950s the majority of sex instruction manuals, published by religious organisations, stressed the moral rather than the physical elements of sexual behaviour, including 'sexual self-control, the primacy of the family, the sanctity of marriage, and the spiritual side of human relationships' (Pearce, 2004: 78–79). Teenage boys were told that masturbation causes 'physiological and moral damage' (Pearce, 2004: 87), that 'sex is a dangerous impulse' (Pearce, 2004: 82) and that they were to abstain from intercourse. What I want to highlight here is the way contraception is never mentioned. Instead asexual purity and purity itself became the 'buzzword of the 1950's' (Pearce, 2004: 87). I also want to draw attention to the aims of these sex education manuals – to shape 'the future man' (Pearce, 2004: 73), conceived of as white, heterosexual, middle-class and Anglo-Saxon-Celtic.

Sex education for young British women in the early twentieth century also aimed to direct women away from promiscuity, identified as unnatural and unclean, and towards virtuous womanhood and healthy motherhood (Bland, 1982). For this reason Bland argues that women were seen as having a duty to fulfil their role as 'guardians of the race' (1982: 372). What is underscored here is the way in which preventative sex education at the turn of the century concerned a particular eugenicist paradigm, one whereby 'parental fitness and responsible breeding' (Bland, 1982: 377) were of special importance, especially for girls who come to bear the moral and racial duty to protect and reproduce the nation's health. As Mort points out, 'social hygiene perpetuated a double standard by insisting that male self-control, though possible, was problematic and that girls should help men to act responsibility by watching their own behaviour' (Mort, 2000: 150). Underlying the emphasis put on girls to regulate male sexuality is a desire to regulate female sexuality.

Not much changes with the advent of sex education in schools. In 1943 the British Board of Education published a pamphlet *Sex Education in Schools and Youth Organisations*. The report noted the need for suitable instruction in schools with parental backing. The content of this report provided the basis for the provision of sex education in secondary schools. The impact of the report has had an enduring effect on school sex education (Hampshire, 2005). Discussing the legacy of the pamphlet Hampshire (2005) addresses sex education policy in England and Wales from the 1940s to the 1960s. He notes that, whilst the 1943 pamphlet officially supported the provision of sex education by schools and youth organisations, it 'did not offer any concrete guidelines of stipulation that such education should be given' nor would the Board 'prescribe sex education classes'. Moreover, the Board 'considered "prior responsibility" for sex education lay with parents' (Hampshire, 2005: 91). According to Hampshire 'this marked the beginning of a strategy of non-decision-making which would continue for the next 40 years' (2005: 91). The policy of non-decision-making is however called into question in the 1950s and 1960s by the British Medical Association. Concerned about the adolescent and health education, particularly in the context of increasing VD rates and fears of adolescent promiscuity, calls were made for a 'comprehensive national policy' so as to improve school sex education (Hampshire, 2005: 95–96). Despite these concerns the government resisted demands for a national policy on the basis it would be an 'illegitimate extension of state activity'. It was left up to the teachers to decide what and how sex education should be taught (Hampshire, 2005: 99). Most teachers were unwilling to challenge the moral agenda promoted in the Department of Education pamphlets such as 'School and the *future* parent' (1956) and 'Moral aspects of the family' (1966) (Hampshire, 2005: 102, my emphasis). This reluctance occurred for a number of reasons: 'general attitudes towards sex, the fear of promiscuity, the attitudes of parents and teachers, and lack of definite leadership from local education authorities' (Weeks, 1989: 256). Hall (2004: 63) cites statistics from 1955 which suggest that five out of six schools did not provide sex education, and, in those that did, the provision was minimal. The sporadic nature of sex education in schools was due to the fact that it was not a mandatory part of the curriculum but determined by the prejudices of local education authorities and head teachers (Hall, 2004: 63). Withholding sexual information from students worked towards maintaining the innocence of children and the category of childhood (Jackson, 1982).

In those schools where sex education was provided the content was a matter of concern. In a study of forty-two books on sex education conducted by the National Secular Society in 1970, the majority were found to be obscure in style, inaccurate in content and badly written (cited in Weeks, 1989: 256). The material used endorsed a conservative view of sex. 'Even the most liberal texts tended to endorse a "stages" view of sexual development, which was either to be happily resolved in heterosexual monogamy or unhappily resolved in sadness and isolation' (Weeks, 1989: 256). What I want to stress in Weeks's account of the stages view of sexual development is the way it produces a chronological model of sexuality, one whereby heterosexuality and the institution of marriage are identified as the final point in becoming a respectable adult.

In her analysis of British sex education Wolpe (1987) further highlights the prominence of this heterosexual moral framework. Wolpe (1987) discusses the legacy of the Crowther Report of 1959 which allocated responsibility to the schools for the 'perceived absence of morality and the failure of families to ensure the correct moral upbringing of their children', especially working-class children (Wolpe, 1987: 39). A key recommendation of the report was that sex education instils a moral order of 'chastity before marriage and fidelity in marriage' (Wolpe, 1987: 39). Wolpe also discusses the Longford Report on Pornography of 1972 which 'condemned what it saw as the reprehensible inclusion of "the more personally relevant sex-education, access to birth control facilities, information and advice on abortion, a sensible attitude to VD"' (Weeks, 1981 cited in Wolpe, 1987: 41). Despite these concerns, numerous studies cited by Wolpe suggest that school sex education provided very little information on birth control, abortion and VD. For instance, a study of five hundred British head teachers conducted by Jackson in the late 1970s found that 'only 10 per cent of schools gave information on contraception and the majority thought this should not be included in sex education' (Jackson, 1978, cited in Wolpe, 1987: 43).

What stands out in Jackson's findings is the way in which adolescent sexuality is framed not so much in relation to the present but rather in relation to *the future*:

> British educators see sex education as preparing adolescents for the future rather than helping them to come to terms with sexuality here and now. Its chief aim, indeed, is apparently to dissuade them from expressing their sexuality at all. (Jackson, 1982, cited in Wolpe, 1987: 44–45)

The lack of contraceptive advice in sex education is considered to be most damaging for adolescent girls as 'it places female sexuality so firmly in the context of marriage and the family' (Wolpe, 1987: 45). Whilst not wanting to dispute the claim that sex education advice involves the silencing and disciplining of adolescent female sexuality (see also Mills, 1992), I want to draw attention to the way in which heterosexuality is constituted as a *future-orientated sexual identity*.

Throughout 1980s Britain a moral framework in sex education prevails. The 1986 Education Act shifted the responsibility for sex education to school governors, who now had control over the content of sex education, and to parents, who had the right to withdraw their children from sex education classes (Durham, 1991; Thomson, 1994: 48). The 1986 Education Act made it clear that sex education should be taught in a context of helping pupils to understand 'the benefits of stable married life and the responsibilities of parenthood' (Weeks, 1981: 295). On the specific question of the provision of contraceptive advice to girls under sixteen, 'the general rule must be that giving an individual pupil advice on such matters without parental knowledge or consent, would be an inappropriate exercise of a teacher's professional responsibilities, and could, depending on the circumstances, amount to a criminal offence' (Thomson, 1994: 48–49). What stands out here is how the provision of information about contraceptives such as condom use to pupils, particularly adolescent girls, becomes criminalised. The policing of the teaching profession was compounded by Section 28 of the 1988 Local Government Act which prohibited any discussion of lesbian and gay relationships in the classroom for fear of 'promoting homosexuality'. Section 28 promoted a moral framework of family life including the benefits of stable married life and the responsibilities of parenthood (Thomson 1994).

AIDS and sex education

The advent of AIDS changed the provision of sex education in the classroom. In 1991 it became compulsory for students aged eleven to fourteen (Key Stage 3) to receive some form of education about HIV and AIDS. The threat of AIDS to public health was recognised as serious enough to warrant changes to the National School Curriculum. Thomson points out that such a move takes a pragmatic approach to sex education. 'Public health pragmatism is concerned to get information to students and to affect their behaviour' (1993: 229). This contrasts, she argues, with 'moral authoritarianism [which] is primarily interested in securing a traditional definition of sexual relations within the educational institution' (1993: 229). The inclusion of HIV education in the National Curriculum was however objected to by conservatives and the religious lobby, who began a campaign for the right of parents to withdraw their children from the classroom (Thomson, 1993: 230). In response to these concerns, the 1993 Education Act established sex education as a distinct subject for all secondary school students in England and Wales unless they were withdrawn by their parents (Thomson, 1994). The initial emphasis placed on public health during this period was thus undermined by a moral authoritarianism (Thomson, 1993).

Governors remained responsible 'for developing the schools approach to sex education in consultation with parents and must ensure that the approach and resources used in the school are consistent with the moral framework' (Thomson, 1994: 53). The moral framework – with its emphasis on marriage and family values – was re-established by making biological reproduction a compulsory element of the national curriculum whilst removing all 'non-biological' aspects, including discussion of STDs and HIV (Lewis and Knijn, 2002: 672). The main reason for removing discussions of HIV/AIDS from the compulsory sex education curriculum 'was because it involved reference to anal sex (even though homosexuality was not explicitly mentioned), which MPs feared would not be accompanied by sufficient moral guidance' (Lewis and Knijn, 2002: 676). Not even the threat of AIDS to adolescents justified teaching them about safer sex. HIV education thus became the responsibility of teachers who were forced to self-censor on issues such as homosexuality and sexual pleasure so as to avoid complaints from parents and governors.

More recently there has been a shift away from limited sex education. The need to inform students about AIDS and STIs and educate them about safer sex 'also made possible discussion of other sorts of sexual relationship and/or activity' (Thorogood, 2000: 434). Yet according to Thorogood (2000: 431) the shift from 'restricted information' to a more 'progressive perspective' 'shares the norms of sexual normativity held by moral traditionalists but feels they are best achieved through open and frank discussion'. So, whilst such a shift in sex education policy may be understood on the one hand to have constituted a loosening of the dominant moral framework, on the other, Thorogood (2000: 434) points out, 'it invoked a desire for more explicit moral regulation', 'more explicit discussion of sexual behaviours, both "normal" and "deviant", and more pervasive forms of control'. 'Since sexual identity in adolescents is not considered "fixed", and therefore, possibly subject to the influence of others, sex education has a duty to be more "morally responsible" as well as more explicit' (Thorogood, 2000: 434). Thorogood's analysis draws attention to the ways in which safer sex education in the classroom increased the regulation of adolescent sexual behaviour. The renewed emphasis on moral regulation occurs because adolescent sexuality is regarded as not fixed but unfinished and malleable. In this way sex education concerns the regulation of an adolescent's *future* sexual identity. Take, for example, the guidelines issued by the Department of Education and Employment in 2000. The new guidelines 'rejected the idea that sex education encouraged teenage sex, stressing the desirability of honest answers and support, at the same time as reiterating the importance of delaying sex and not "teaching" homosexuality' (Lewis and Knijn, 2002: 684). Whilst New Labour policies are considered to mark a departure from the strict moral rhetoric of the late 1980s and early 1990s and reflect a more positive approach to sex education, I want to suggest that the emphasis placed on the benefits of delaying sex and not 'teaching' homosexuality involves the production of a future-oriented adolescent (hetero)sexual subject.

Thomson and Blake (2002) trace a further shift in the language and policy of English sex education in the late 1990s. Under the New Labour government the concern is not the moral effects of sex education on adolescents but 'effectiveness defined in terms of outcome, both behavioural (falling teenage pregnancy rates, less unsafe sex, later first sex) and cost effectiveness' (2002: 188). According to Thomson and Blake (2002: 189) this shift in policy from morality to effectiveness is worrying since interventions which focus on outcome target 'at risk' or 'risky' individuals and disadvantaged communities. Targeting information about condom use to specific groups, they argue, mirrors the punitive and stigmatising sexual health policies of the US, policies which I discuss below. What is required is the continuation of a policy of 'universal entitlement and an ethos that sex education should contribute towards self-awareness and "intimate citizenship" as well as behaviour change' (Thomson and Blake, 2002: 189), a policy which I evaluate towards the end of the chapter in relation to the Australian context where sex education on HIV/AIDS has been part of the school curriculum in many states since 1992.

Condom wars

During the second part of the twentieth century the content and ideology of North American sex education undergoes some significant changes. The sexual conservatism in the early twentieth century, with its emphasis on the family and the nation, is replaced in the 1960s and 1970s with sexual liberalism and an emphasis on freedom of choice in such areas as 'sexual orientation, pornography, and unmarried minors' access to contraception' (Moran, 2000: 195). The forces behind these shifts are identified by Moran as the sexual revolution of the 1960s and the Sexual Information Education Council (SIECUS), with its leanings towards sexual libertarianism (Moran, 2000: 195). Moran also identifies the women's liberation movement together with the development of a visible homosexual rights movement in the 1960s as having had an impact on the liberalisation of sex education. Together these broad-ranging social changes constitute a historical shift in the lives of American adolescents away from a focus on sexual self-control and chastity before marriage which 'was losing its privileged position as the sole site for sexual relations' (Moran, 2000: 198) and towards a space of sexual experimentation and innovation (D'Emilio and Freedman, 1997: 264). What characterises this changing ontology of adolescent sexuality in the 1960s is the 'affirmation of sexual pleasure and the acceptance of a public world of youthful dating' (D'Emilio and Freedman, 1997: 274). In addition, D'Emilio and Freedman identify the contraceptive revolution with its separation of procreation from erotic expression as questioning 'not only the primacy of marital sex but also the primacy of heterosexuality itself' (1997: 274).

But by the end of the 1970s a conservative reaction against women's liberation, gay rights and adolescent sexual practices takes place (Moran, 2000: 203). The backlash was fuelled by conservative critics who seized upon statistics of increasing abortion rates to argue that the availability of contraception in the 1970s was not having a positive impact on adolescent lives:

> Activists resurrected the old charge that *the availability of sex education, contraception*, and abortion all actually *encouraged adolescent sexual activity* – and pointed out, accurately, that rising rates of intercourse between unmarried adolescents in the 1970s had indeed proceeded alongside the increased availability of contraception and abortion and the broader dissemination of sex education. (Moran, 2000: 203, my emphases)

What is clear here is the direct link between the provision of sex education including information about contraception such as condom use and the incidence of premarital sexuality. These concerns came to play a big role in Ronald Reagan's electoral victory of 1980. With a renewed emphasis on sexual restraint, conservatives mandated against the sexual liberalism of the 1970s. In 1981 Congress passed legislation which came to be known as the Chastity Act. The act denied funds to programmes or projects that provided abortions or abortion counselling and mandated abstinence education in the sex education it did fund (Moran, 2000: 204). Withholding funding to programmes that do not promote the message of abstinence continues to dominate US policies. In 2003 President Bush declared he would spend $15 billion on global AIDS relief. Receiving aid under the programme has 'moral strings attached' such as the promotion of abstinence over condoms (Vasagar and Borger, 2005: 1). This has had a disastrous effect in Africa, particularly in Uganda where the rapid decline in the distribution of condoms has resulted in a significant increase in rates of HIV infection (Vasagar and Borger, 2005: 2). What I want to draw out here is the ways in which funding for HIV health education programmes involves the policing of the condom.

In the mid-1980s the prominence of AIDS funding for adolescence changes the shape of sex education in the US classroom. The money allocated to the problem of adolescent AIDS and HIV education 'replaced altogether the broader kinds of sexuality education that would include discussions of sexism, homosexuality, and ethical values' (Moran, 2000: 208). The adolescent AIDS crisis 'narrowed the parameters of the sex education debate' and restored 'a fear of disease to a central position in sex education' (Moran, 2000: 210). The question in the 1980s was no longer whether schools should *offer* sex education but what *kind* of sex education they should present. Sex education became geared towards the enforcement of 'a stricter chastity among unmarried youth' (Moran, 2000: 213) and a conception of 'sexuality and adolescence primarily in terms of danger' (Moran, 2000: 216).

The conception of adolescent sexuality in terms of danger is most apparent in the 1990s. During the period 1989 to 1999 there was a sharp decrease in the discussion of condoms in classrooms as effective in preventing HIV and other diseases. Much of the critique of condom use came from Christian right research institutes that infiltrated sexuality research and produced misleading statistics and data on condoms. 'Conservatives charged that there are tiny (five micron) holes in condoms that sperm are too big to penetrate but through which the HIV virus could pass' (Irvine, 2002: 116). Alongside this there was a proliferation of misleading information on condom use such as the claim that 'when you use a condom, it is like playing Russian roulette. There is a greater risk of a condom failure than the bullet being in the chamber' (Irvine, 2002: 121). By comparing the practice of safer sex to Russian roulette and by citing medical journals which claimed that condoms have holes in them conservatives were able to claim that comprehensive sex education programmes were dangerous to youth.

The circulation of misleading sexual knowledge on safer sex was not the only way in which the condom became targeted in debates on adolescent sexuality. What was just as significant, if not more so, argues Irvine (2002), were the debates on sexual speech in the classroom, including discussions of gay sexuality and attempts to educate youth on condom use.

> By the mid-eighties, opponents of comprehensive sex education escalated their claims about the performativity of sexual speech. They continued to argue that sex education caused young people to engage in sex, but they also rhetorically fused speech and action to allege that speaking sexuality in the classroom is tantamount to 'doing it'. Sex education they charged *is* sexual abuse. (Irvine, 2002: 133)

Irvine makes two key points in regard to sex education in the US post-AIDS. First, the accusation that speaking about sex produces sexual behaviour is equivalent to the charge 'that sexual speech affects, and constructs sexual identities. The fears, of course, travel in one direction – that by talking about homosexuality, otherwise heterosexual youth will be seduced into it' (2000: 63). There is of course little concern that no-sex education constructs heterosexuality as compulsory. Second, 'simply talking about lesbian/gay issues in the schools constitutes child abuse' (2002: 64). Irvine suggests that the real basis for the opposition to discussing homosexuality alongside non-stereotypical gender roles concerns the fear that talk of sex would 'disrupt normative heterosexuality' (2002: 172) with young people being converted to homosexuality 'through positive role modelling' (2002: 173).

According to Irvine what lies at the heart of these claims about the performativity of sexual speech as sex *and* sexual abuse is the historical definition of childhood. Battles over sexual speech – what not to mention in the classroom, i.e. sex, safer sex, condoms, sexuality – derive from the ideal of romantic childhood and the nation's ideal of children's vulnerability and the need to protect children. 'By definition the romantic child's innocence depends on protection from sexuality – shielded from all information and knowledge' (Irvine, 2002: 13). No-sex education is thus legitimised on the basis that it protects children from knowledge of sexuality and in so doing protects the nation's health. A policy of promoting not knowledge of safer sex but the ignorance of knowledge (Sedgwick, 1990) therefore concerns the regulation of sexuality. According to Sedgwick ignorant effects can be 'harnessed, licensed and regulated on a mass scale – especially around sexuality, in modern Western culture' (1990: 5). And at the same time she points out that unknowing is a privilege which has disproportionate disciplinary effects, effects which I discuss later in the chapter in relation to the policy of *targeting* (safer) sex education to certain groups of youth.

On one level the success of promoting an ignorance of knowledge via the abstinence-only curriculum lies with its claims to protect the category of childhood. As Levine puts it, 'abstinence connects powerfully to that deep parental wish: to protect and "keep" their children by guarding their childhood' (Levine, 2002: 109). But on another level, I want to stress that the Christian right campaign against comprehensive sex education is not so much about a parental wish to keep children in a state of childhood as about protecting the *future of the adolescent*. As Levine points out, 'believing that teen sex is a form of self-destruction, the abstinence-only people (who are also anti-choice activists) ask kids to "choose life", not necessarily their current lives but better lives *further down the road*' (2002: 106, my emphasis). What I am seeking to highlight here is the way abstinence-only sex education claims to protect kids not so much from themselves, in terms of the present, but rather a *future which is yet come*. Abstinence educators point kids '*towards* something worth having' (Levine, 2002: 106). Within this narrative the condom serves as a threat towards a future conceived of as heteronormative.

But is it the case that the condom disrupts the narrative of (hetero)sexuality. Does the condom threaten kids' futures? In his account of the cultural narrative of futurity in political discourse

Edelman (2004) argues that it is no coincidence that the future is condensed into the figure of the child. Moreover, Edelman suggests that the survival of the social order is secured in the Imaginary form of the child. 'We are no more able to conceive of a politics without a fantasy for the future than we are able to conceive of a future without the figure of the child' (Edelman, 2004: 11). In Edelman's analysis of the rhetoric of futurity in contemporary culture he draws attention to the human cost of conceiving citizenship in relation to claims about 'the child as futurity' (2004: 31) as opposed to the lived experience of real children. At the same time he argues this futurity requires queerness as its figurative outside. Queerness constitutes a threat not so much to heterosexuality but to the future and the realisation of the future. 'Queerness for contemporary culture ... is understood as bringing children and childhood to an end' (Edelman, 2004: 19) '*Queerness* names the side of those *not* "fighting for the children", the side outside the consensus by which all politics confirms the absolute value of reproductive futurism' (Edelman, 2004: 3). Edelman's analysis draws attention to some of the problems faced by sex educators in the US. On the one hand his analysis suggests that comprehensive sex education is so demonised and pathologised precisely because sex talk and talk of condoms in the classroom threaten to disrupt the heteronormative logic of reproductive futurism. But on the other hand Edelman's analysis questions the view of many sex educators who position the condom as protecting adolescent sexuality and the nation's health. What I am seeking to highlight here is the way knowledge of safer sexual practices in comprehensive sex education also concerns a reproductive logic in that it positions the condom as protecting the future life of an imaginary child and an about-to-be-realised (hetero)sexual citizen.

Condoms, adolescence and futurity

To address the extent to which the condom is implicated in the regulation of the adolescents future, let's consider the US policy of targeting safer sex education to specific 'risk' groups (see also Irvine, 2002). In addressing the question of why some North American adolescents do not use condoms Moran suggests 'a student's response to education is itself *socially determined*'

(2000: 222, my emphasis). Moran (2000: 222–223) identifies social background and socio-economic status as a measure of an adolescent's ability to process classroom knowledge of safer sex effectively. Middle- and upper-class kids, he argues, respond more positively to information about condom use. Since 'young people of higher socioeconomic status are more *oriented toward the future* than their less advantaged peers, they may be more likely to change their behaviour in response to new knowledge ... To students who *lack this future orientation*, who find the question of where they will be in five or six years a matter of fatalism or indifference, an education based on future consequences has little meaning' (2000: 223, my emphases). Thus, according to Moran knowledge of condom use has little impact on poor kids because they lack a future-oriented subjectivity.

But is this the case? Patton (1995a) draws attention to the effects of targeting sex education to certain 'disadvantaged' youth. She argues that the policy of targeting HIV education on condom use to the 'at risk' teen, identified as either gay or a member of the black or Latino urban underclass, categorises the white heterosexual middle-class adolescent as normative by associating HIV only with certain embodied others. 'Deviant bodies – one racial and one homosexual – ... constitute the visible boundaries of the "normal" adolescent by both inscribing and being inscribed by their need to have "knowledge" of safe sex' (Patton, 1995a: 346). Hence, unlike Moran, Patton's analysis draws attention to the ways in which disadvantaged youth are *positioned* by the condom as unable to achieve a future-orientated adolescent sexual subjectivity since their bodies are considered 'intrinsically physical and unlikely to change their behaviour' (Patton, 1995a: 354).

What stands out in Patton's account of the differences between the deviant non-heteronormative Other and heteronormative adolescent self is the way the condom excludes 'youth of colour' and 'gay teens' from a narrative of futurity. The policy of targeting safer sex education to certain youth identified as troubled and troubling sexual bodies positions these bodies as incapable of becoming adolescent. What I am seeking to highlight here is that the passage from childhood into adolescence and finally adult (hetero)sexuality is thwarted by *the need to know* about the condom and the practice of safer sex:

> The basic logic of separating the young deviant from the 'normally abnormal' adolescent (thereby determining *who needs to know about safe sex*) depended on the construction of normal adolescence as a passage from a precultural body (the innocent child) through a civilizing process (the disembodied adolescent with desires unfulfilled by practices) to sexually responsible adulthood (i.e. monogamous, married, procreative, white, heterosexual). Two deviations from this development tale were envisioned: *black bodies* never passed through the cultural, having neither adolescence nor civilized adulthood. Similarly, *homosexual bodies* passed into adolescence, but emerged into a distinct subculture in which real (heterosexual) adulthood was foreclosed. (Patton, 1995a: 339, my emphasis)

This account nicely illustrates how the condom stops time and stops adolescence. Further still, Patton's analysis illustrates how the condom in the context of safer sex education is the figurative outside of reproductive futurism. For black and gay kids the condom constitutes a narrative of non-futurity. But at the same time the condom is constitutive of a narrative of preservation and planned reproductive futurity for middle-class white adolescents.

My point is further illustrated in Patton's (1998) discussion of two Christian sex education websites targeted at teens in the early 1990s. In her account of the home pages of 'True love waits' sponsored by the Southern Baptist Convention and 'Wait trainer', a home page on the Christian web domain integrityol, Patton describes how 'both sites argue that most teens are not even having sex, or rather most middle-class white teens are not' with 'Wait trainer' claiming 'that unplanned pregnancy is the domain of the poor' (1998: 365). What is most striking in Patton's account of 'True love waits' is not just the promotion of abstinence but also the way young people who take the 'abstinence challenge' are asked to sign 'convenant cards' that read: 'Believing that true love waits, I make a commitment to God, myself, my family, my friends, *my future mate, and my future children* to be sexually abstinent from this day until the day I enter a biblical marriage relationship' (1998: 365, my emphasis). Here then there is no mention of condoms. Neither is there, as Patton points out, any mention of homosexual practices. The health message 'to put a condom on your heart' differentiates white middle-class adolescents from poor teens who are described as not being able to wait.

In making a promise to be sexually abstinent for the sake of my *future* mate and my *future* children the adolescents who wait become future-oriented heterosexual citizens responsible not so much for the protection of their own sexual health but for unborn future generations.

In many ways Patton's account of safer sex education carefully draws attention to and problematises the universalist assumption of an adolescent subjectivity. However, in her analysis of the developmental process Patton appears to take for granted the category of white heterosexual middle-class adolescence as normative. Reflecting critically on her own deconstructive method, Patton (1995b: 179) has suggested that this legibility of the self through the inscription of the 'Other' is somewhat limited in that it presumes 'the constitution of a "self" through reverse discourse in too unified a manner, a manner that insists too strongly on the bipolar structure of subject-constitution that is required within the self-other model'. In an attempt to avoid such a bipolar account of subject formation Patton (1995b) addresses the interrelation between bodies and space. In responding to Patton's concerns I want to highlight the interrelation of objects and time and in particular the object of the condom and the temporality of adolescence as significant for understanding the social process of becoming a sexual subject and the ontology of adolescent sexuality post-AIDS. Turning my attention to the Australian context where talk of condoms in the classroom has been encouraged, I point out the formation of an adolescent subjectivity takes place not through an ignorance of knowledge but via knowledge of *condom use*. In my analysis I seek to highlight that being an adolescent in the Australian context is tied not so much to the stigmatised bodies of the Other who are constitutive of the normative self but rather the object of the condom as an extension of a future-oriented white, middle-class (hetero)sexual subject.

Safer sex education

In 1992 AIDS education became a mandatory part of secondary state school education in New South Wales. Secondary state schools were expected to take responsibility for teaching students about HIV/AIDS. Whilst the Australian school curriculum is controlled at the state level, with each having its Department of School Education, the Australian federal government made funding available for curriculum development and service training in order to build the capacity of teachers to undertake HIV/AIDS and sexuality education (Lupton and Tulloch, 1996). The aims and objectives of this sex education curriculum are to teach students not just about HIV/AIDS but also safer sex and the skills to negotiate condom use so that adolescents can make 'behaviour change related to personal development and health status' (Lupton and Tulloch, 1996: 254).

Lupton and Tulloch point out that the AIDS sex education policy document 'privileges "knowledge" incorporating both information and understanding as the key to achieving responsible and fulfilling sexual expression. The programmes are aimed at developing a heightened self-consciousness [and] a better understanding of the sexual self' (1996: 254). In comparison to the US, the Australian model is identified as libertarian in that it asserts 'that personal freedom and self-knowledge can only be achieved through the free expression of one's sexual proclivities and desires' (Lupton and Tulloch, 1996: 253). At the same time, following Foucault, Lupton and Tulloch recognise the ways in which adolescent sexuality is constructed and regulated by the discourses and practices of sex education. Students are taught 'technologies of the self that work towards shaping and disciplining the body in certain ways, normalizing it according to assumptions about the ideal body' (Lupton and Tulloch, 1998: 22). What stands out in their account of the disciplining of the adolescent body in the Australian sex education curriculum is the way it concerns not just the 'unfinished body' but also the *object of the condom*. For instance, there is a privileging of 'the body that is able to manage sexual desire, sensibly protecting itself against unwanted advances, sexually transmissible diseases and pregnancy' (Lupton and Tulloch, 1998: 22). What I am seeking to highlight here is how the 'the process of becoming a sexual body' (Lupton and Tulloch, 1998: 22) and indeed 'being' an unfinished adolescent involves *knowledge about condom use.*

The promotion of condom use in comprehensive HIV/AIDS school-based sex education can thus be understood within a Foucauldian framework as concerning the normalisation of adolescent sexuality. Indeed, in their analysis of the unfinished adolescent body Lupton and Tulloch draw on Foucault's (1979) account of sex education 'as a strategy for the construction of "normal" and "responsible" sexuality, a means of regulating and normalizing young people in encouraging them to take up forms of sexuality that have been deemed acceptable' (Lupton and Tulloch, 1998: 266). But in so doing they query Foucault's account of power in relation to HIV/AIDS education. They do so with reference to social research conducted in 1993 with 138 senior high school students (sixteen- and seventeen-year-olds) from metropolitan and regional government schools in New South Wales. The focus of Lupton and Tulloch's study was students' experiences of HIV/AIDS and sexuality education. From their empirical data they find that HIV/AIDS education and sexuality education tend 'to be regarded as lacking' (Lupton and Tulloch, 1996: 266). More specifically, Lupton and Tulloch find that school-based educators are reluctant 'to be specific about safer sex techniques, such as the use of condoms', and there is no provision of condom vending machines in schools (1996: 258). Lupton and Tulloch therefore surmise that 'little impression was gained from students' accounts of their HIV/AIDS and sexuality classes that the apparatuses of governmental power were successfully working to *constitute their sexual personae in defined ways*' (Lupton and Tulloch, 1996: 266, my emphasis).

But is this view accurate? Do the students' concerns regarding the lack of information about safer sex techniques, such as condom use, indicate that the school-based sex education has failed to constitute students sexual identities in defined ways? I want to suggest that this view is a little premature. My reservation is based on Lupton and Tulloch's (1996) observation that for some of these students 'school-based education often tended to downplay the nature of adolescent sexuality, preferring to pretend that students were *not yet* sexually active' (1996: 258, my emphasis). The view that adolescents are not yet sexually active indicates that sex education is framed within a narrative of futurity, a sexuality which is yet to come. What I want to draw attention to here is the way knowledge of the condom constitutes this yet to be realised (hetero)sexuality.

This matter of condoms and futurity is also evident if we consider the impact of sex education programmes promoting condom use in the Scottish context. Whilst the responsibility for sex education in England and Wales lies with school governors, in Scotland local education authorities are still responsible for the sex education curriculum. This has changed somewhat with the Scottish Executive and the 2000 package on sex education. Although the new package developed some clear guidelines, Buston, Wight and Scott (2001) point out that 'guidance has not been prescriptive, with each school developing its own programme, if it chose to'. As a consequence 'room for variation has been wide. There has been no consistency, either, in who is responsible for developing sex education programmes within a school' (Buston, Wight and Scott, 2001: 354). In an attempt to examine the utility of school sex education for young Scottish women and men, particularly in relation to the content of sex education lessons and its influence on sexual behaviour, Buston and Wight (2002, 2006) conducted a large trial of sex education. Twenty-five secondary schools from the east of Scotland participated in their sex education trial. Some of these schools agreed to be allocated randomly to deliver the sex education program SHARE (Sexual Health and Relationships) to secondary three and four pupils aged between fourteen and sixteen, whilst the other schools were to continue with their existing sex education. As sex education is not mandatory in Scotland and parents are in some instances consulted about the content of programmes, Buston, Wight and Scott (2001) found existing sex education to be varied in its delivery, content, depth and provision. 'Common features were the emphasis on taking responsibility and a harm reduction approach, although the extent to which schools wholeheartedly endorsed this varied' (Buston, Wight and Scott, 2001: 356). By contrast 'central to the [SHARE] programme are sessions specifically intended to influence behaviour: to develop sexual negotiation skills using interactive video, a role-play session developing skills to say "no", and a "condom skills" session on obtaining and correctly handling condoms' (Buston and Wight, 2002: 234–236).

Through their research Buston and Wight (2002, 2006) examined the impact of the SHARE package on students' ability to learn about sex. They found that young women had generally positive things to say about their skills-based sex education. 'Specifically, the young women valued: being shown different kinds of contraceptives, being told how effective each is, how to obtain/plan to use them with one's partner, and/or how to use them (in some cases having a chance to put a condom on a model phallus)' (Buston and Wight, 2002: 240). For the majority, who were not yet sexually active, knowledge about condoms was described as useful in the *future* (Buston and Wight, 2002: 245, my emphasis). Although young men felt that 'sex education had come too late because by that time they "knew it already"' (Buston and Wight, 2006: 142) changes in *future* male behaviour included 'carrying a condom at all times; using a condom; knowing how to use a condom properly ... and feel[ing] more confident about communicating with women, especially in relation to *persuading them to use a condom*' (Buston and Wight, 2006: 145, my emphasis). In this context (safer) sex education not only constitutes (hetero)sexuality as future oriented, it also impacts on the matter of consent and condom use, issues which I explore in greater detail in Chapter 7.

Despite my concerns that safer sex education produces a future-oriented adolescent (hetero)sexual subject, the narrative of the unfinished adolescent body is one that need not end. This point is stressed by Lee (2001: 78) in his account of childhood and good education in the twenty-first century. Lee suggests that, with the educational change arising from the use of information and communication technologies, school students are no longer positioned as docile bodies or indeed becoming bodies 'on their way to completion, to a finished state of adulthood' (2001: 77) but in processes of 'becoming without end' (2001: 78). If we are indeed constitutionally unfinished and human life involves not so much the body but the extensions we are living through, the challenge for sex educators and social scientists is to be open to the possibility of the condom as an extension of young people themselves, issues which I address in Chapters 6 and 7.

3

Condoms and sex research

What are the consequences of getting adolescents to speak about the condom and their sexual experiences in the public arena? What impact has sex research had in producing knowledge of adolescent sexuality? In answering these questions this chapter seeks to provide a history of sex research on the condom. The object of my analysis is government-funded sex research on adolescence. Focusing on HIV/AIDS research conducted within university departments throughout the 1990s, I address the role social scientists have played in constructing knowledge about the condom and sexuality post AIDS. The aim of the chapter is to question the research methods used by social scientists to evaluate adolescent sexual behaviour and condom use. In particular, I analyse the consequences of qualitative research methods and their impact on the construction of adolescent sexuality. My concern in this chapter is not the content of condom stories (see Chapters 6 and 7) but the production of safer sex narratives. In examining research on condom use I show how the issue of gay and lesbian invisibility raised in relation to the 'Rubber Wars' in Chapter 1 concerns the production of safer sex stories. In particular, I seek to highlight how qualitative methods constitute adolescence as an unfinished, yet to be complete (hetero)sexual identity, one that is narrativised via the condom.

Researching sex from the 1960s

The sociologist Julia Ericksen has documented the manner in which social scientists in the US in the mid-twentieth century employed scientific methods, especially statistical methods, during times of sexual crisis in order to gather information for the purpose of developing effective public policies. Sex researchers, according to Ericksen, are not neutral figures but active participants in the production of knowledge. 'Because the researcher holding the hypothesis selects, words and orders the questions, questionnaire design is particularly vulnerable to researcher bias' (Ericksen, 1999: 9). What interests Ericksen is not just the bias of the sex researcher or indeed the funding of specific research topics but the changing assumptions and concerns about sexuality in sex research. 'The assumptions driving the research helped create the sexuality the research revealed' (Ericksen, 1999: 11). Tracing these changes, she argues, reveals the history of sexuality in the twentieth century. In what follows I address what this history looks like in the second half of the twentieth century paying particular attention to the significance of the condom in the production of adolescent sexuality.

During the early 1960s sex researchers in the US were cautious about surveying the sexual behaviour of youth. 'Researchers who asked what students were doing sexually could be accused of promoting promiscuity' (Ericksen, 1999: 72). By the mid-1960s, and with the rise of student protest and its presumed relationship to sexual revolution, there is an increase in the number of sex surveys targeted specifically at college students. Researchers aimed to examine 'the extent of change' (Ericksen, 1999: 77) and did so via questions about sexual permissiveness including questions about sexual intercourse before marriage and its frequency. Few studies even mentioned contraceptive use. Middle-class college students provided accounts of premarital intercourse as normative, especially amongst women, thus confirming the view of the sexually permissive 1960s. Ericksen points out that, whilst these findings are interpreted as a reflection of social change, 'the pro-sex attitudes of many researchers undoubtedly contributed to these changes' (Ericksen, 1999: 85).

The perceived permissiveness of the 1960s comes under question in the research of the sociologists Gagnon and Simon. In their sex surveys they find little evidence to support the claim that a sexual revolution is taking place. By comparing their findings, taken from questionnaires with North American high school students, to Kinsey's findings taken from eighteen thousand interviews conducted during the 1940s and 1950s, Gagnon and Simon discover little change in sexual behaviour. They find that 'rates of early and premarital coitus had remained stable over time and were still largely a function of courtship' (Ericksen, 1999: 80). In switching their focus from adults to adolescents Gagnon and Simon (1970) make some interesting sociological observations about adolescent sexual behaviour. Addressing the relationship between social change and sexual behaviour, they suggest that the social has a direct impact on the sexual. More specifically, they argue that sexual behaviour and sexuality are created by society and learnt from social scripts. The content of these scripts, found in pornography, women's magazines, advertising and even the publication of sex surveys changes over time and varies in different cultural context. In positing sexual behaviour as scripted behaviour Gagnon and Simon's rationale for doing sex research becomes one of measuring not so much sex itself but the sociocultural context in which sexual behaviour is learnt. Scripted behaviour is regarded as particularly apparent in relation to adolescence, a period where 'training in the postures and rhetoric of sexual experience is now accelerated' (Gagnon and Simon, 1970: 30). Scripted behaviour marks the beginning of adult sexuality and a break with what went on beforehand.

Whilst Gagnon and Simon's research on sexual behaviour questions the received wisdom of sexual revolution, the explosion of sex surveys conducted on North American high school students in the early 1970s 'made student sexual behaviour seem like a break with society rather than a product of it' (Ericksen, 1999: 81). According to Ericksen, sex surveys 'almost single-handedly created the social problem of adolescent sexuality' (Ericksen, 1999: 90). Throughout the 1970s Ericksen finds that sexual activity amongst adolescents was 'taken for granted in surveys, and its consequence was assumed to be pregnancy' (1999: 102). Sex researchers addressing (the presumed) sex lives of early adolescents focused on girls, with teenage boys left out of surveys. But, by ignoring boys, surveys assumed that male sexuality was 'all-consuming and uncontrollable' and thus suggested that their 'sexual urges were unchanged and unchangeable' (Ericksen, 1999: 97). And, in targeting girls, researchers assumed that teenage pregnancies were a female event and unintended, thus characterising these girls as victims in need of protection. 'Few asked young women how they became sexually involved or whether they wanted to, and none asked if they enjoyed it'

(Ericksen, 1999: 99). Questions about consent were absent or secondary and figured only briefly in research findings.

Ericksen's analysis of the history of the North American sex survey exposes two underlying assumptions on the part of researchers. First, an assumption of heterosexuality and, second, within this privileging of heterosexuality an assumption that sexuality is a property of gender. Sex researchers viewed 'women's desire for men as a natural part of being a woman and men's desire for women as a natural part of being a man' (Ericksen, 1999: 223). They also viewed the male sex drive as different from, and stronger than, the female sex drive (Ericksen, 1999: 12). What concerns Ericksen is that young women as a group 'had historically been talked at and not listened to' (1999: 109), especially in relation to their experiences of sexual pleasure, desire and negotiation. What particularly troubles Ericksen about sex research is the way consent 'has yet to become a methodological concern' (1999: 222). Ericksen draws attention to research findings from an unusual study undertaken in 1987 which did include two questions on non-voluntary intercourse. 'Two thirds of those who became sexually active at age 14 or younger described nonvoluntary sexual intercourse as did half of those who started at age 15' (Ericksen, 1999: 107). According to Ericken these findings indicate 'that many sexually active teenagers might indeed be victims, but in a quite different sense than previously imagined. Their victim status could *not be cured by condoms*' (Ericksen, 1999: 107, my emphasis). Ericksen's comment raises some important questions about the role of the condom in relation to adolescent sexual practices. Her observation that the condom cannot solve the problem of non-voluntary adolescent sexual practices raises the question of condom use and consent, issues which I explore in greater detail in Chapter 7.

Researching sex in the 1990s

Whilst a major function of the condom in the 1970s and early 1980s was to stop teenage pregnancy, by the end of the decade sex surveys helped shift the meaning of the condom to 'a panacea for AIDS' (Ericksen, 1999: 191). In the context of AIDS sex surveys aimed to encourage behaviour change towards the use of condoms. In surveys of gay men the message from researchers was 'not simply that gay men *must use condoms* but that they must change from a deviant lifestyle to one modelled on heterosexual marriage. Lesbians in the meantime were ignored' (Ericksen, 1999: 226, my emphasis). By contrast, in AIDS-related surveys of (heterosexual) adolescents researchers '*encouraged the use of condoms*' (Ericksen, 1999: 228, my emphasis). According to Erickson these surveys reassured young people that their own sexual desires and preferences are normal. What I want to highlight here is the way heterosexuality is normalised via the condom. This is evidenced in the way sex researchers differentiate between homosexuals who are obliged to use condoms and heterosexuals who are encouraged to do so.

During the late 1980s and early 1990s a number of small-scale surveys were funded to measure heterosexual AIDS transmission. Sex researchers who had previously ignored the incidence of HIV amongst gay men were now interested in whether AIDS was a danger to all North Americans, including heterosexual men. Even though little evidence supported the assumption that heterosexuals, especially heterosexual teens in the US, were at risk of HIV, in 1988 the Federal Centre for Disease Control (CDC) began a series of health risk surveys among high school students, which asked questions about sexual activity, and knowledge of HIV risks (Ericksen, 1999: 191). In 1989 eight thousand high school students were interviewed using the same questions. Ericksen argues that by not recognising the empirical fact that gay men at the time accounted for most of the young adult cases of AIDS in the US, social scientists played a key role in the process of creating the myth of heterosexual transmission, and prioritising school students over gay men in sex research.

> A few researchers acknowledged the lack of concrete evidence that AIDS was spreading among the young and the heterosexual, and some studies of youth emphasised other STD's as much as AIDS. But all used AIDS to justify their research, and none pointed out that teens did not have especially high risks of contracting the disease. (Ericksen, 1999: 191)

The bulk of the CDC's funding went to surveys of all students – not to those minority youth truly at risk – with white middle-class students receiving the most attention. Sex researchers focused on middle-class students on the basis of the assumption 'that only they had the time or education to achieve sexual bliss' (Ericksen,

1999: 12). The focus on middle-class adolescents assumes that they respond more positively to sex education and have the capacities to minimise sexual risk in the context of AIDS. In this chapter I examine some of the consequences of these assumptions and the impact they have had in producing knowledge of class and racialised differences.

Attempts in the early 1990s to conduct large-scale US national surveys on adolescent sexual behaviours which lead to AIDS were, however, opposed by Congress. Two surveys proposed to ask questions about vaginal intercourse, oral intercourse and anal intercourse and thus didn't assume sex was heterosexual. But it was the plan to include boys and ask them if they had had male sexual partners which received the most opposition. Discussing this opposition Ericksen (1999) points out there was a fear that boys might become homosexual from the survey. The fear was of the behavioural consequences of talk about sex. 'Conservatives believed surveys would inform young people of things they might not know and tell the more knowledgeable that such behaviour was permissible' (Ericksen, 1999: 203). Ericksen points out the surveys were also blocked by conservatives because of the potential for undesirable results such as the possibility that a significant proportion of the population was actually gay. Despite this opposition, in 1992 a National Survey of American adults took place. The findings, published in a popular text, *Sex in America*, portrayed Americans in a more conservative light. Heterosexual marriage was found to be alive and well. Most Americans had few sexual partners or extramarital affairs and practised monogamy. Hardly any respondents reported having same-sex sexual experience, homosexual erotic desire and a homosexual identity, with only a small percentage of the men in the sample identified as homosexual. In questioning this very limited picture of homosexuality in America Ericksen draws attention to the problem of knowledge production particularly as it is shaped by the sex researchers' views of the world. Whilst Ericksen's account focuses on the problems of researcher bias in producing normative sexual knowledge, in the next section of this chapter I examine the significance of *research methods* in privileging and normalising heterosexuality. I do so by considering how different sex research methods have impacted on individuals understandings of their sexual selves and their sexual practices in the context of AIDS.

Sex research methods

The question of research methods is addressed by Poovey (1998) in her account of *Sex in America*. In her analysis of the quantitative methods used in the National Sex Survey Poovey considers the impact of statistical data in producing a particular story of sex at odds with both the permissive 1960s and the existence of gays and lesbians. Her main concern is that statistical methods of knowledge production work towards the making of normative social categories of people, constituted for the purposes of description.

> Statistical analysis does impose certain limits on the kinds of things that one can study; or phrased differently, statistics demand that what can be studied be represented in a certain way. Most basically ... one can only develop statistics about entities that can be counted, or phrased differently again, in order to analyze something – like sexuality – statistically, one must represent it so that it seems amenable to quantification. (Poovey, 1998: 386)

In deploying quantitative methods, sex researchers represent an inefficient and limited picture of sexuality and sexual behaviour as discrete, and unchangeable. This occurs because the survey reduces sexual identity to sex acts. To represent sexuality in this way is to 'represent sex – or certain sex acts – as amenable to administration, in that it – or they – can be vilified if they do not conform to what the majority represents as "normal"' (Poovey, 1998: 388). Statistical knowledge, according to Poovey, is then internalised by a silent majority 'driven by the desire to be normal and to know that they, and their sexual behaviours are normal' (1998: 374). Statistical knowledge is thus normative in that it 'inspire[s] people to govern themselves in keeping with the common good' (1998: 385).

Whilst the definitive account of sexuality in *Sex in America* presents heterosexuality as a statistical norm, 'homosexuality defies quantification' (Poovey, 1999: 387). This is the case, argues Poovey, because homosexuality 'does not produce external signs and because, even when it does, these signs may not refer to the kind of stable essence essential to counting' (1998: 387). Poovey suggests that 'even if the government had given the sex researchers money, they could not have produced knowledge about the group that an AIDS-related survey might well have wanted to target: gay men and lesbians' (1998: 387). What are required are 'new knowledge practices' (1998: 390) since 'statistical analysis is not sufficient for understanding sexuality because, in turning sexuality into sex, statistics create the false impression that such social behaviour can be addressed simply and in isolation from the social matrix in which they are embedded' (1998: 392–393). In capturing the social context of sexuality, non-statistical research is understood to break with a definitive characterisation of homosexuality and heterosexuality. In the context of AIDS, Poovey argues, such research is imperative since empirical studies are well placed to address 'why so many American youths continue to think of unprotected penetrative sex as the only "real" sex, even though they know the risk of AIDS' (1998: 391).

In order to deal with the problem of sexual knowledge in the era of AIDS Poovey suggests we develop critical accounts of how the knowledge-producing instruments employed by institutions like governments or universities create some kinds of knowledge and foreclose others. At the same time Poovey calls for new modes of knowing about sex and imagining intimacy that depart from normative understandings of sexuality. In addressing Poovey's suggestions I want to question her claim that statistical analysis alone is responsible for the production of normative accounts of sex and sexuality whilst other methods of researching sexuality can facilitate knowledge of gays, lesbians and non-normative heterosexualities. By critically analysing *qualitative* sex research methods I seek to question the assumption that non-statistical methods break with the characterisation of homosexuality and heterosexuality as discrete and oppositional categories. What I am looking to highlight is how *qualitative* methods also produce knowledge of heterosexuality whilst foreclosing knowledge of others.

In the British context the sociologist and social historian Liz Stanley (1995) analysed the effects of the research methods deployed in the 1990 National Survey of Sexual Attitudes and Lifestyles. The survey was originally supported by the state. Funding was, however, withdrawn at the last minute by Margaret Thatcher, who refused the use of public funds to conduct the survey. It finally went ahead in 1990/91 with the financial support from the Wellcome Trust. Almost eleven thousand sixteen- to fifty-nine-year-olds throughout Britain took part in the survey. The findings were later published in *Sexual Behaviour in Britain* (Johnston, Wadsworth, Wellings and Field, 1994). The survey aimed to gather information about '"sexual attitudes and lifestyles" – that is, about what is happening sexually at the moment – so that it can then act as a baseline for discerning and measuring *future* change in the area of sex and sexuality' (Stanley, 1995: 234, my emphasis). The main objective of the survey was to prevent HIV/AIDS. Many of Stanley's criticisms of the survey reflect the concerns of Ericksen and Poovey. For instance, Stanley notes the assumption of sexual and social change and questions the process of measuring it. 'Defining what constitutes "sexual change", and exploring why it might occur, deciding how to measure it, and discerning when it is happening, are individually and collectively, not simple matters' (Stanley, 1995: 233). Although the survey did not assume that all sex is necessarily heterosexual, Stanley notes that there was an attempt to characterise Britons as having a particular lifestyle 'conceived as heterosexual or, for a tiny minority, gay male, with lesbian "lifestyles" being too numerically insignificant even to be discussed' (Stanley, 1995: 60). Despite the inclusion of a range of sexual practices, Stanley suggests that what is missing from the survey are questions relating to sexual meanings, emotions and feelings, issues which are crucial to understanding sexual behaviour, 'for the same sexual act can mean different things and so can be experienced differently' (1995: 234).

What stands out in the 1990 National Survey is the invisibility of gays and lesbians in the survey data. According to Stanley (1995) this is not a true reflection of sexuality in Britain but rather a result of the research process itself. The problem of invisibility is both a consequence of the interview question schedule and the conduct of the interview. Whilst the survey interview, with its emphasis on confidentiality, anonymity and non-judgemental questions was seen to encourage a feeling of trust between interviewer and respondent, the survey's methodological approach and assumptions produced an under-representation of non-heterosexual sexual behaviour, with just over 1 per cent of British men and 3.5 per cent of men living in London identified as involved with a same-sex partner and a tiny 0.3 per cent described as having had lesbian sexual experience. This under-representation of gays and lesbians is attributed to the privileging of heterosexuality in the ordering of the questions, an ordering which positions gay experience as problematic, thus discouraging the disclosure of gay and lesbian experience. The under-reporting of gay male experience is also attributed to a refusal by gay men to participate in the planned interviews (Keogh cited in Stanley, 1995: 51–52). In an earlier study, carried out by Project Sigma, half of the gay men asked whether they would participate in the National Survey said they would refuse (Stanely, 1995: 51). Stanley discusses the reluctance of gay men to self-disclose taboo or stigmatised sexual practices outside of a safe gay subcultural context:

> For many, probably still most, gay people, central to self-perception of being gay is precisely an absence of self-disclosure except in certain highly specific and safe social contexts and with only very particular persons, while the National Survey makes the assumption that a two hour interview with a stranger will successfully enable such consequential self-disclosure. (Stanley, 1995: 1)

AIDS social research

HIV/AIDS research dealing specifically with the gay community has been much more effective in dealing with the problems of self-disclosure. In the Australian context the social researchers Kippax and Kinder (2002) discuss the successes of AIDS research from a 'gay informed' standpoint, one employed at the National Centre in HIV Social Research at the University of New South Wales in Sydney. Research conducted in this gay-informed context involves a critical understanding of the researchers' own assumptions about gay sex and homosexuality and a take-up of the research participants' understanding of homosexuality and homosexual practice (Kippax and Kinder, 2002: 98). Engaging in a gay-informed standpoint therefore avoids any negative characterisations of gay sexual behaviour and gay sexuality. It does so by shifting the focus away from the individual behaviours of gay men to a broader social context in which sexual practices gain meaning in relation to pleasure, intimacy, love and risk (Kippax and Kinder, 2002: 97). In so doing sex researchers have been able to provide more effective analyses of their data. For instance, Kippax and Kinder found the practice of unprotected sex –

without a condom – to be negotiated within the context of existing relationships. Such a strategy has been defined and has come to be understood in HIV/AIDS-related sex research as negotiated safety (Kippax and Kinder, 2002: 100). The significance of such research is that it opens up an exchange between social scientists and health promotion in ways that enable the issue of unprotected sex within relationships to be addressed (Kippax and Kinder, 2002: 101).

The benefits of exploring gay sex in sex research are further elaborated in the work of Gary Dowsett, an Australian sociologist. In his text *Practicing Desire* Dowsett suggests that attempts made by social scientists to understand the history of gay life in the context of HIV/AIDS must avoid objectifying homosexuality and in particular avoid 'the notion that sodomy equals homosexuality' (1996: 33). The problem lies with HIV/AIDS researchers who 'collect huge data sets on sex practices with scant regard to sexual meanings or pleasures'. How often, he asks 'are respondents ever asked what it felt like?' (1996: 33). On the one hand Dowsett is critical of a scientific or positivistic approach in social research which reduces the configuration of the sexual to individual sex preferences. 'It is this lack of the relational character of sexual activity, the inattention to sexual meanings and their creation, an ignorance of the social constituents and contexts of sexual activity, which deprives much research of the answers so urgently required' (1996: 35). But on the other hand Dowsett is equally critical of attempts made by sex researchers to decouple sodomy from homosexuality via 'the development of a non-sexuality-specific notion of *high risk practices*' (1996: 33). As he sees it, the categorisation of gay-community-identified men, men who have sex with men and heterosexual men or men who have sex with women also amounts to a reductionist model of sexuality based on individual preferences (1996: 34). 'The dilemma for the researcher is to inquire deeply and rigorously into the operation of desire without abstracting it, on the one hand or making it concrete on the other' (1996: 35).

What really troubles Dowsett with the shift in focus from anal (gay) sex to high-risk practices in sex research is a de-homosexualisation of HIV/AIDS. In the attempt to defuse homophobic responses he argues that 'homosexual transmission of HIV becomes a simple variation in a unitary domain of *male* sexuality' (1996: 34). The consequences of such a focus on male sexuality include the obliteration from view of the struggles of gay communities with HIV, and further still it 'ignores the subordinate position of homosexuality and the struggle of gay men (and lesbians) to resist the structural relation between heterosexuality and homosexuality' (1996: 34). According to Dowsett the problem of heterosexism is compounded by the deployment of gender in social science research addressing male sexuality, a conceptual category that privileges heterosexuality and has little to offer for understandings of gay sex and desire he finds in a series of life history interviews. Dowsett is equally critical of theoretical analyses of sexuality, particularly deconstructive accounts produced by queer theorists, in their ability to adequately illustrate the doing of sex and the desiring sexual body in qualitative research data. These accounts, he argues, rob the body of sex.

Dowsett's methodology foregrounds the relationship between sexual activity and meaning. He is interested in the social interactions and sensations of gay sex (1996: 37). As a sociologist he seeks to understand the experience of sexual engagement in relation to issues of choice, action and resistance (1996: 42). For Dowsett, sociological research 'recognizes that history and culture produce and shape the potentials and constraints within which individuals live their lives' (1996: 40). Whilst Dowsett's interest in the historically constructed experience of gay life in the context of AIDS clearly highlights the benefits of deploying qualitative methods, I want to stress that the use of other post-structural methods may be particularly useful in illustrating how heterosexism and heteronormativity operate in relation to social research on HIV/AIDS. My interest in analysing qualitative methods is to address the impact of being asked to talk about safer sex. In what follows I seek to highlight the ways in which the safer sex story as told by adolescents produces knowledge of (hetero)sexuality. In so doing I illustrate how heterosexuality is privileged in AIDS research on adolescents and condom use.

Speaking of condoms

Since the 1980s, and in the context of AIDS, new sexual stories have been created. According to Plummer 'a striking set of new stories are emerging around "safer sex"' (1995: 158). Stories of safer sex including condom use have disrupted the dominance of the old narrative of procreation. In its place 'a new language of sexual experience is in the making which shifts emphasis away from the traditional tale of penis-vagina procreational sex' (1995: 159). Addressing the 1982 publication by New York gay men *How to Have Sex in an Epidemic*, Plummer points out that the term 'safer sex', with its emphasis on bodily pleasure without the exchange of body fluids, has also 'shifted the languages and stories through which we understand the complexities of our sexualities and politics' (1995: 160). In discussing this shift Plummer recognises the impact of the women's movement of the late 1980s as having produced a change in sexual narratives of the erotic which break with 1970s anti-sex feminist stories (see Chapter 5 for an analysis of this historical shift).

Whilst these stories are understood to involve the proliferation of new sexual practices, AIDS, he argues, is a major narrative that is not just about sex. In documenting the moment at which new AIDS stories emerge Plummer is less interested in what people say than in the significance of these stories in their own right, as topics to investigate. Plummer avoids seeing these stories as mere facts of our sexual natures or indeed the truth about sex. He also avoids seeing human stories as mere texts that need to be analysed and instead sees stories 'as *social actions embedded in social worlds*' (Plummer, 1995: 17). 'They have conservative, preservative, policing control tasks – as well as transgressive, critical, challenging tasks' (Plummer, 1995: 176). Plummer does not therefore take the telling of sexual stories for granted and recognises that some stories cannot be told. Moreover, Plummer addresses the social conditions which have enabled the emergence of new stories in the late twentieth century. The issue for Plummer concerns not so much the content of stories but how these stories come to be told and heard. Like Ericksen, Plummer argues that sex research stories do not merely reflect our sexual lives but play an active role in their construction. Social research is part of the activity whereby people tell stories about themselves and the broader world around them. Plummer is also interested in the producers of research. He refers to them as 'coaxers, coachers and coercers' who 'probe, interview and interrogate' and in so doing 'can play a crucial role in *shifting the nature* of the stories that are told' (1995: 21, my emphasis). Plummer is particularly interested in the consequences of saying a particular story under particular circumstances. For Plummer matters of consequence are crucial in story analysis. In asking the question 'what does a certain kind of story play in the life of a person or a society', he replies 'sexual stories lay down routes to a coherent past, mark off boundaries and contrasts in the present and provide both a channel and a shelter for the *future*' (1995: 172, my emphasis).

Plummer's analysis clearly highlights the performative social dimension of sexual stories. What I want to draw out from Plummer's account of sexual stories is the question of consequence. What are the consequences of saying the safer sex story? How should we interpret these stories? How should we analyse them? What are the consequences of young people being asked to talk about safer sex and especially condom use? Do these stories mark time in the present and provide a channel and shelter for the future? What impact have the provokers of safer sexual stories had in relation to young people's understanding of themselves in the context of AIDS? Has sex research enabled the telling of a particular sexual story whilst foreclosing others? To what extent do these stories change our conception of adolescence? To begin to answer these questions I turn to Fraser's (1999) account of the telling of sexual stories:

> Stories about one's (sexual) practices (and fantasies, desires, etc.) are told and recounted (in more or less literal or intentional ways) *in order that the self may perceive itself (and be perceived) to 'have' a particular identity*. Hence although Foucault does not refer to sexuality *itself* as a technique of the self, insofar as sexuality is often – through narrative – constructed as a problem upon which the self consciously reflects, and a practice which is carried out by the self ... sexuality might itself be understood to be just such a (narrative) technique. (Fraser, 1999: 20–21, my emphasis)

If stories of sexual practices are told so 'that the self may perceive itself (and be perceived) to "have" a particular identity', the safer sex story should not therefore be interpreted literally, that is, as tellings of the truth of the condom and as a measure of an adolescent's response to health campaigns promoting AIDS awareness. In other words, addressing the history of sex research in the context of AIDS involves not a consideration of *what* condom stories tell 'us' about the impact of the object on the everyday lives and the intimate views of young sexual citizens but rather *how* the telling of contemporary safer sex stories concerns a 'technique through which the individual is rendered (and renders itself) intelligible' (Fraser, 1999: 19). If one of the consequences of sex research is that it constructs sexuality as a narrative technique of the self, what role have sex researchers played in this process? What impact has the condom had in rendering the adolescent intelligible as having a *particular* sexual identity? What does the embedment of the condom in the safer sex narrative reveal about the history of the condom? According to Harre (2002: 25) 'an object is transformed from a piece of stuff definable independently of any story-line into a social object by its embedment in a narrative'. If this is the case, how does the transformation of the condom into a social object in AIDS research impact on the history of sexuality? To address these questions I turn to empirical studies of safer sex.

AIDS research, condoms and adolescence

Since the early 1990s there has been a proliferation of social science research on safer sexual practices and the impact of AIDS educational advertisements promoting condom use. What is most apparent regarding this body of empirical research is how it has focused on adolescent experiences. Much of this work has involved small-scale qualitative as well as quantitative research projects on adolescent sexual practices and adolescent attitudes towards national AIDS public health education campaigns including government-funded mass-media campaigns, and secondary school sex education (see Chapter 2). As mentioned previously, Poovey claims that social research could provide new modes of knowing and imagining intimacy and desire which break with the characterisation of heterosexuality and heterosexuality as distinct sexual identities. Poovey also suggests that social methods are particularly important for addressing the problem of unsafe sex and youth. Poovey anticipates that qualitative methods could question the normalisation of heterosexuality and the invisibility of gays and lesbians in statistical analysis. But is this the case?

During the 1990s qualitative research undertaken in the UK aimed to measure and assess adolescent sexual behaviour and in so doing effectively contribute towards government policy on

HIV/AIDS education. Funding for research was primarily geared towards studies of heterosexuality. Research on adolescent girls in England carried out by Holland, Ramazanoglu, Sharpe and Thomson (1998) addressed how gender impacts on young people's heterosexual behaviour and the problems of condom use. The benefits of such research according to Thomson (1994: 54) is that 'qualitative research that has explored the ways in which young men and young women understand sex and sexuality and the way in which they relate to dominant ideals of masculinity and femininity provides an alternative empirical basis from which educational initiatives can develop'. Research on young heterosexual men from Scotland conducted by Wight (1993a, 1994a, 1994b, 1996) addressed the specific impacts of masculinity and class on young men's ability to understand the term 'safer sex' and practise heterosex with a condom. These studies along with the research findings are analysed in greater detail in Chapters 3, 6 and 7. What I want to highlight here is the assumption in these studies that condom use is problematic for heterosexual adolescents, particularly for young heterosexual men. In other words, buried within these research projects is a normalisation of unsafe sex. The researchers assume that unsafe sex – without a condom – is characteristic of adolescent (hetero)sexuality.

During the 1990s there was also a proliferation of studies on adolescent sexual behaviour in the Australian context. Most of the research was undertaken in order to assess the uptake of safer sex and examine the factors which both encouraged and inhibited behaviour change towards condom use. The Research Centre for Sex, Health and Society (previously known as the Centre for the Study of Sexually Transmissible Diseases) at La Trobe University, Melbourne, has over the past two decades produced a diverse range of statistical knowledge on the sex practices of Australian adolescents including high school students and university students, as well as students from non-English-speaking backgrounds (see Chapter 4). In 1997 the Centre conducted a nationwide survey of 118 government secondary schools. Lindsay, Smith and Rosenthal (1997) gathered data from 3550 questionnaires to assess the knowledge, attitudes and practices of secondary high school students in years ten and twelve. Many of the survey questions related to issues of sexual activity and condom use, and asked questions related to last sexual experience (with or without condoms), knowledge of HIV, perceptions of risk in relation to HIV and STDs, levels of casual sex, communication about condoms during last sexual encounter, reasons for the non-use of condoms, ability to negotiate condom use and students' beliefs about peers' condom use (Lindsay, Smith and Rosenthal, 1997). The 1997 National Schools Survey aimed to 'detect changes over time at a national level in young people's HIV/STD-related knowledge, attitudes and practices' (Lindsay, Smith and Rosenthal, 1997: 11). One question in the survey asked students about their current feelings of sexual attraction and whether they are attracted to people of their own sex, opposite sex or both sexes. The question was absent in the previous national survey conducted in 1992 (see Dunne *et al.*, 1993). Whilst the addition of this question may be regarded as positive in that the researchers are not assuming heterosexuality, the bulk of the questions privilege heterosexuality. What I want to draw attention to is how the privileging and indeed normalisation of heterosexuality in this survey takes place in relation to questions not about unsafe sex but rather about safer sex, that is, *condom use*.

The normalisation of heterosexuality via the condom also appears in social research undertaken in Australia. Qualitative research conducted by Lupton and Tulloch aimed to measure the effectiveness of HIV information in popular media, news reporting and sex education in providing an adequate source of HIV/AIDS knowledge for secondary students (Tulloch 1992; Tulloch and Lupton, 1997; Lupton and Tulloch, 1996, 1997, 1998 (see Chapter 4 for an analysis of this research). Here I want to focus on the implications of Lupton and Tulloch's (1998) study on the 'unfinished adolescent' in HIV/AIDS sex education. As mentioned in the previous chapter, their research included a series of discussion groups with sixty-five boys and seventy-three girls from five schools in metropolitan Sydney and four in New South Wales in their penultimate year of secondary schooling. These focus groups were conducted in order to explore the 'concept of the "unfinished body" as it is understood and experienced by Australian adolescents in the context of HIV/AIDS' (1998: 24). Lupton and Tulloch find that young people desired 'more "in-depth" information about HIV/AIDS and other sexually transmitted diseases' (1998: 24–25) which is not bogged down in academic jargon-ridden language. Such in-depth knowledge concerned the physical experience of HIV/AIDS, 'what it actually does to your body' (1998: 25). In the discussion groups students talked about the ways in which school-based education tended to 'beat around the bush', 'not get down to earth', 'not get to the point' and glossed over issues 'without exploring them in depth' (1998: 27). They wanted 'to hear stories of people with HIV/AIDS, and to be able to talk more freely with others about sexuality and AIDS' (1998: 29). At the same time, Lupton and Tulloch acknowledge that getting adolescents to talk about sex has certain social consequences, as they point out in their direct reference to Foucault (1978).

> Speaking about children's sex, inducing educators, physicians, administrators, and parents to speak about it, *causing children themselves to talk about it*, and enclosing them in a web of discourses which sometimes address them, sometimes speak to them, or impose canonical bits of knowledge on them, or use them as a basis for constructing a science that is beyond their grasp – all this together enables us to link an intensification of the interventions of power to a multiplication of discourse. (Foucault cited in Lupton and Tulloch, 1998: 23, my emphasis)

Yet Lupton and Tulloch do not recognise the role that *social researchers* play in causing school kids to talk about sex. In other words, they fail to grasp the consequences of their own qualitative research in enclosing the body of the unfinished adolescent in a web of discourses around sexuality. They thus underestimate the social effect of getting high school students to talk about AIDS education and safer sex to social researchers. This is surprising given that they draw on Foucault's account of the confession as 'a form of surveillance and normalization, whether it is young people "confessing" their thoughts and feelings to each other, or to parents, doctors or teachers' (1998: 30) but they do not consider their own research in this way.

Furthermore, in addressing the discourse of the 'unfinished adolescent body' in AIDS school-based sex education Lupton and Tulloch do not take into account the significance of their research in producing knowledge of adolescents as *'unfinished sexual beings'* (1998: 23, my emphasis) in the process of becoming sexual beings. In other words they take for granted and thus normalise the category of the unfinished adolescent. In a deconstructive account of adolescence Gordon cautions against conceptualising adolescence as unfinished or as he puts it 'a utopian site of a free-floating "liminal" exploration of myriad nonbinding identifications and desires' (1999: 6). Gordon is also critical of research on adolescence and suggests this must be resisted for two reasons. First and foremost, the project of the unfinished adolescent body treats 'adolescent experience as something empirically available "in its own right"' (Gordon, 1999: 6). Second, and more importantly, such discourses 'mask the extent to which heterosexuality is privileged in the discursive construction of adolescence' (Gordon, 1999: 6). The narrative of adolescence in the discourse of the unfinished sexual body configures adolescence as a temporal category. Here sexuality is figured in terms of 'an immanent futurity, that which the subject *will* acquire – the present of adolescent is ubiquitously structured by an adumbrated future' (Gordon, 1999: 6). In respect to the subjectivity attached to the unfinished adolescent body 'heterosexuality will be constantly invoked, but its realization will be constantly delayed' (Gordon, 1999: 10).

If adolescent subjectivity *is* intelligible, but as Gordon points out this intelligibility is 'grounded in a narrativistic mode of knowledge' (1999: 6), then AIDS research appears to invoke a narrativised mode of knowledge production of which Gordon is so critical. From Gordon's analysis we may therefore make a number of conclusions regarding AIDS research on adolescence. First, the empirical categories invoked by such research, such as the 'unfinished adolescent body', figure adolescence as a sexual category which is geared towards the not too distant future. Second, this body of research invokes a narrativisation of adolescence, one which naturalises heterosexuality as an imminent futurity. What this chapter has drawn attention to is the role played by AIDS researchers in the production of adolescence as a future-oriented (hetero)sexuality. This is witnessed in the way the safer sex story now counts as acceptable social scientific knowledge about adolescent sexuality. Moreover, I have shown how the condom itself produces a narrative of delayed (hetero)sexuality. If the condom marks time and is constitutive of adolescent subjectivity, from this we could conclude that the condom has indeed become a social thing embedded in the narrative of heterosexuality. Whilst this chapter has drawn attention to the consequences of adolescent safer sex stories, in the following chapter I seek to examine further the ways in which for some young people condoms do not connote or constitute movement from the present to the future.

4
Safer sex representations

Sex research and sex education in the context of AIDS have extended beyond the classroom. In response to the AIDS crisis of the 1980s the Australian and British governments funded national public health television campaigns. The aim of these advertising campaigns was to promote AIDS awareness and safer sex practice to the general heterosexual population. Since then there has been a proliferation of safer sex representations in the mass media. These mainstream AIDS representations have been studied and analysed in order to assess their effect on individual awareness and behaviour change, particularly for adolescents. What lies at the heart of these analyses is the impact of safer sex representations in the construction of sexuality. Altman points out that the media is central to understanding the new public visibility of the condom and sexuality.

> The globalization of world culture, with new messages carried across national boundaries by television and radio, has meant an expansion of what in the 1970s seemed a particularly American form of sexual consumerism. Before we denounce such developments as irresponsible, it is important to note that they have been accompanied by large scale promotion of 'safe sex': *the condom*, as much as the sex club or the videos of Madonna, *has become an emblem of sexuality in the modern world*. (Altman, 1995: 105, my emphases)

Altman's reading of the promotion of safer sex suggests that the condom has both global and national significance as an 'emblem of sexuality'. In this chapter I examine the large-scale promotion of the condom in the US, UK and Australian mass media from the mid- to late 1980s. The focus is on AIDS representations on television and in popular advertisements. I do so with particular reference to the Australian 'Grim Reaper' advertisement together with audience research studies on this national AIDS awareness campaign. In so doing I seek to highlight the ways in which the condom has come to define national identity, sexual citizenship and the production and recognition of difference.

The Grim Reaper campaign

I am taking the 1987 'Grim Reaper' television advertisement as my main object of analysis because of its significance as the first national media campaign to produce knowledge of AIDS in the Australian context. Even today Australians who were children at the time of its broadcast vividly remember the sixty-second commercial as a distinctive moment in the history of AIDS. The $3.5 million advertising campaign was produced by the National Advisory Council on AIDS and was funded by the Commonwealth government. It took place over a two-week period during April of 1987. The specific aim of the campaign was to promote safer sex to heterosexuals. The popularity of this campaign, especially the figure of the Grim Reaper, has been noted in AIDS research (Bray and Chapman, 1991; Crawford *et al.*, 1990; Lupton and Tulloch, 1996, 1997; Rigby *et al.*, 1989; Tulloch, 1992). According to Lupton (1994) the advertisement's popularity is generated by its 'controversial' depiction of AIDS.

> The terrifying figure of the Grim Reaper, swathed in swirls of mist, is shown aiming a bowling ball at collections of people, all dressed to represent white, respectable and healthy 'middle-Australia' (the women in dresses, the men wearing shirts and ties). These figures are set up like bowling pins and then are all knocked over by the giant bowling ball, and finally are shown lying as if dead. Images include a little girl crying in fear as the bowling ball comes rolling towards her and a baby being knocked from its mother's arms as both are bowled over by the giant ball. The Grim Reaper then raises its arm in a victory gesture and bares its teeth in a grisly smile, celebrating its 'strike'. The closing shot of the advertisement show a collection of Grim Reapers all busily engaged in their game of knocking over people with bowling balls, suggesting the proliferation and rapid spread of AIDS. The accompanying voice-over, a deep and sonorous male voice, warned the audience that 'if not stopped, [AIDS] could kill more Australians than World War II. But AIDS can be stopped, and you can help stop it'. Audiences were

then exhorted, 'If you have sex, have just one safe sex partner, or always use condoms – always'. (Tulloch and Lupton, 1997: 40)

For Tulloch (1989) the image of the Grim Reaper conveys a message to the Australian general public that '*everybody* (including the privileged but defenceless mother and child) is at risk from this death' (1989: 105).

> The audio message that accompanies the advertisement 'have sex with a regular partner or use a condom always' also works to 'shock heterosexuals into the realization that everyone, not only homosexual men and intravenous drug users, were at risk from contracting HIV and dying of AIDS'. (Lupton, 1992: 13).

> The voice-over of the 'Grim Reaper' advertisement emphasized that members of the audience, (hailed as 'you'), can 'help' stop [AIDS] by having 'one safe partner' or using a condom in every sexual encounter. However, this message of personal responsibility and agency jars with the images of the advertisement that depicts the random nature of death from AIDS and the passivity of the victim. (Lupton and Tulloch, 1997: 41)

The message of safer sex targeted at the general population is understood to have decreased homophobic constructions of AIDS in the media. According to Lupton 'press accounts of AIDS upon gay lifestyles diminished in favour of the threat posed by the disease to multipartnered heterosexuals' (Lupton, 1993: 319). In producing a shift in the meaning of AIDS, from an association with the 'Other' (Lupton, 1992: 14) to 'the risk of HIV infection to the entire Australian sexually active population' (Lupton, 1993: 308), the 'Grim Reaper' advertisement is understood to have diminished 'the "gay plague" as a dominant metaphor' (Lupton, 1991: 73).

The heterosexualisation of AIDS

In the British context, Weeks (2000) and Berridge (1996) point out a parallel shift in the history of AIDS representations. Between 1983 and 1986 Weeks (2000) notes that the tabloid press defined AIDS as a homosexual disease. The category of 'homosexuality' served as the Other 'whose presence served to define what is normal in the rest of the population' (Weeks, 2000: 145). In attaching AIDS to the lifestyle of the homosexual, gay men become defined as deviant and guilty victims whilst heterosexual transmission is seen as innocent and ignored.

But by the mid-1980s the initial stereotyping of AIDS as a gay plague in the British media diminished. This shift was largely the result of two national television campaigns, the 'Iceberg' and 'Tombstone' advertisements, which were broadcast between late 1986 and early 1987 as part of the British Government's AIDS public health campaign. The Iceberg campaign featured the word AIDS as an iceberg with the tip of the letter A above the water, demonstrating that the levels of AIDS in 1987 are just the tip of the iceberg. A voiceover accompanies the advertisement:

> There is now a deadly virus that anyone can catch from sex with an infected person. But you can't always tell if someone is infected. The people who have died so far will be the tip of the iceberg. So protect yourself; it's safer if you use a condom. And remember, the more sexual partners, the greater the risk.

The 'Tombstone' advertisement begins with a volcano erupting; you then see a man carving the word 'AIDS' into a tombstone. The stone then falls over and a copy of the 'AIDS: don't die of ignorance' leaflet which accompanied the campaign, and was posted to every household, drops on to the stone, along with a bunch of lilies, to represent death. A voiceover accompanies the advert:

> There is now a danger that has become a threat to us all. It is a deadly disease and there is no known cure. The virus can be passed during sexual intercourse with an infected person. Anyone can get it, man or woman. So far it's been confined to a small group, but it's spreading. So protect yourself, and read this leaflet when it arrives. If you ignore AIDS it could be the death of you. So don't die of ignorance.

According to Berridge the representation of AIDS 'as a threat to us all' and the focus on prevention in the advertisement normalised the disease. The medium of television, she argues, was critical in the 'mainstreaming' of AIDS in Britain during the mid-1980s (1996: 130).

The £7.5 million Iceberg and Tombstone television advertisements, together with the distribution of the leaflet 'AIDS: don't die of ignorance' to 23 million British homes, are understood to have constituted a 'distinct and unusual period of perceived national crisis' and more specifically as a period of 'wartime emergency' (Berridge, 1996: 7). 'AIDS was officially established as a high-level national emergency, as a national crisis on a par with the Falklands or the Second World War' (Berridge, 1996: 7). Not since the 1940s propaganda campaigns against venereal disease had such a level of funding by public broadcasters been seen (Berridge, 1996). In promoting safer sex to the nation, television broadcasters established notions of 'national community and national interest rather than public interest' (Berridge, 1996: 113). The condom appears central to this process as the advice to 'protect yourself: it's safer to use a condom' is presented to the nation as a whole.

Whilst the propaganda campaign of 1987 is understood to have normalised AIDS as a threat to the heterosexual population and marked a shift away from the British media's construction of AIDS as a gay plague, Watney (1994: 19) points out that the campaign 'AIDS: don't die of ignorance' entirely ignored the social group most devastated by HIV, gay men. Watney is especially critical of the secondary advice that accompanied the 'AIDS: don't die of ignorance' leaflet: 'Anyone can get it, gay or straight, male or female. Already 30,000 people are infected. At the moment the infection is mainly confined to relatively small groups of people in this country. But it is spreading'. According to Watney the message 'intended to dismiss the majority of people with AIDS as members of a relatively small group of people' (Watney, 1994: 20) thus effectively de-gaying AIDS. The campaign drew crucial resources away from the group that most needed it – young gay men. The redirection of funding to the general population and the subsequent ban on discussing gay and lesbian sexuality in the classroom (via Clause 28) had the adverse effect of increasing the stigma attached to gay men and lesbians, a stigma Watney argues was particularly harmful to gay youth in terms of both identity formation and much-needed information about safer sex.

Whilst the disassociation of homosexuality from HIV/AIDS on network television is understood to de-gay AIDS, this disassociation is also perceived to refigure 'homosexuality' as dangerous and diseased (see Treichler, 1988; Landers, 1988: 282; Fuqua, 1995: 202; Vance, 1994: 108; Gott, 1997: 147). According to Williamson (1989) the representation of 'AIDS as a monster' does not produce a connection between AIDS and heterosexuality, but does the opposite, it creates a *connection* between AIDS and homosexuality. AIDS 'claims, chooses, rages, and kills with all the senseless yet directed energy of a mad axe murderer' (Williamson, 1989: 74) and yet the monster 'is precisely "unacceptable" sexualities' (Williamson, 1989: 77). This is particularly evident in the 'AIDS carrier' story, a story that Watney suggests 'belongs to a cluster of similar stories, well known from popular fiction and film, about vampires, mysterious killer-diseases, dangerous strangers, illicit sex' (Watney, 1992: 153). 'The male homosexual becomes an impossible object, a monster' (Watney, 1987: 77). If, as Watney and Williamson point out, the image of the monster is constitutive of other 'dangerous strangers', 'illicit sex' and 'unacceptable sexualities', does the figure of the Grim Reaper on Australian national television consequently re-gay AIDS? How are we to understand the production of sexuality in relation to the 1986 Grim Reaper campaign?

According to Lupton, the portrayal of 'AIDS is Heterosexual' (Lupton, 1993: 324) in the 'Grim Reaper' advertisement takes place via the killing of 'ordinary Australians' (Lupton, 1991: 71), particularly women and children, represented as vulnerable, potentially contaminating, and as at risk in relation to HIV/AIDS:

> It was not until the 1987 government sponsored 'Grim Reaper' AIDS education campaign, with its emphasis on heterosexual sexual activity as a risk behaviour for HIV infection, that the *figure of the woman with HIV/AIDS became overt in mass media portrayals of HIV/AIDS*. The 'Grim Reaper' television advertisement featured several women as the 'ten-pin' victims of the bowling ball thrown by the image of death, including a young woman holding a baby and a little girl. (Lupton, 1996: 100, my emphasis)

> Instead of ten-pins, a collection of stereotypes representing the diversity of 'ordinary' Australians were knocked down (killed) by the huge bowling ball aimed by the figure of Death. These included a housewife, a baby, a little girl and a footballer. (Lupton, 1992: 13)

In many ways Lupton's account of the 'feminine AIDS body' in the Australian context converges with other analyses of mainstream AIDS representations in the US and UK during this period (see Gilman, 1988; Tulloch, 1989; McGrath, 1990; Juhasz, 1990; Singer, 1993; Treichler, 1992). The description of a threatened, vulnerable blonde woman with baby and the figure of the child being bowled over and killed by the bowling balls delivered by the Grim Reaper in the public space of the bowling alley resonates with Singer's (1993) analysis of the logic of sexual safety in the US during the 1980s. According to Singer the family 'is being repackaged as a prophylactic social device', 'as a strategic and prudential safe sex practice' (Singer, 1993: 85). Films such as *Fatal Attraction* represent private domestic space and monogamous and marital heterosexuality as 'safe' by displacing anxiety about sexual risk and danger 'onto the presence of women, especially women who occupy non-traditional roles' (Singer, 1993: 186). According to Treichler the circulation of stereotypical images of white heterosexual women in AIDS representations as 'the whore', 'innocent victims' and the 'madonna' (1992: 42) 'fuels a conservative agenda for women – marriage, family children' (1992: 51). At the same time they 'reinforce the incorrect message to women of color and others that they are *not* at risk' (1992: 43). The contradictory message to women that they are safe, vulnerable and potentially dangerous rehabilitates traditional heterosexuality and challenges 'the very gains of the women's liberation movement: economic, political and sexual independence' (Juhasz, 1990: 27–28). What these analyses highlight is the regulation of women's sexuality in the era of sexual epidemic.

Gilman's (1988) historical analysis of AIDS representations in the US in the late 1980s illustrates a similar theme. Gilman refers to a cartoon of mid-March 1987 which appeared in the *San Diego Tribune* and presented the source of heterosexual AIDS in the form of a group of prostitutes represented as a threat of death. According to Gilman such a representation parallels the history of the iconography of syphilis in the nineteenth century whereby 'a new group is labelled as a source of disease, women – but not of course all women, only those that are beyond the social pale of respectability' (1988: 269). The stigmatisation of women's bodies in AIDS representations isolates those with the disease and at the same time 'limits the "majority's" anxiety about their own potential risk' (Gilman, 1988: 269). Whilst Gilman's account draws a strong parallel between the historical past and the present, his analysis takes a different direction to that of Treichler, Juhasz and Singer. More specifically, Gilman's history of the representation of sexually transmitted disease – as concerning the categorisation of the diseased as Other – forecloses a closer examination of the regulation of gender and (hetero)sexuality in AIDS representations.

Despite these limitations, historical accounts of AIDS which look to the past highlight a significant theme in images of contagion, contamination and sexuality. For instance, in Brandt's account of the representation of sexually transmitted diseases he too draws attention to the visibility of women's bodies (Brandt, 1987: 191–192). Brandt refers to posters designed for US servicemen from the Second World War which depict women with venereal disease, many of which feature pictures of 'loose' women and prostitutes. In one poster, the face of a pretty woman appears next to the warning 'She may look clean – But. Pick-ups, "Good time" girls, prostitutes spread syphilis and Gonorrhoea. You can't beat the Axis if you get VD.' The warning is for men to avoid sex not just with prostitutes but also casual sex with 'loose women' in order to defend the nation and Europe as a whole. This depiction of venereal disease in the mid-twentieth century parallels McGrath's (1990: 147) account of a 1988–89 English public health AIDS advertisement. In the two-page advertisement, which features a full-page photograph of an attractive woman, the accompanying text reads 'If this beautiful woman had the virus which leads to AIDS, in a few years she could look like the person over the page'. On the next page the exact same photograph appears with the comment 'Worrying isn't it'. The representation of a healthy, sexually attractive, white woman with AIDS pathologises women as 'reservoirs of disease: as degenerate and dangerous'. According to McGrath the image of beauty is a mask that conceals all that is rotten.

A further historical parallel between these two adverts is the way they appear to be addressed to a heterosexual male audience who must protect themselves from attractive, desirable women. In the AIDS advertisement part of the printed text at the bottom of the page states 'having fewer partners is only part of the answer. *Safer sex also means using a condom*, or even having sex that avoids penetration. HIV infection may be impossible to recognise, but it is possible to avoid' (my emphasis). This message is similar to Brandt's account of the preventative public health policy during the Second World War whereby 'as many as fifty million condoms were sold or freely distributed each month during the war' (Brandt, 1987: 164). Providing condoms to troops marked an important reversal of First World War military policy and constituted an implicit recognition of the inability of officials to control the troops' sexual drives (Brandt, 1987: 164).

What I want to draw attention to in the era of AIDS is how the audience for condom advertisements changes. For instance, the Iceberg and Tombstone television advertisements in the UK and the Grim Reaper campaign in Australia target women as well as men. Moreover, during the mid-1980s many mainstream US magazines – including women's magazines such as modern *Bride*, *Vogue* and *Family Circle* – start to advertise condoms to women. In order to reach a female audience the condom undergoes a 'makeover, from sleazy to "smart"', a strategy which 'involves desexualizing the condom' (Gamson, 1990: 273). This desexualising strategy was triggered in the US by a multimillion-dollar advertising campaign which included the promotion of Mentor condoms. Discussing an advert for 'Mentor' condoms Treichler (1987: 222–223) illustrates the historical shift in the targeting of condoms to female consumers. In a full-page colour advertisement an attractive healthy white woman looks pensively out at the camera: 'I never thought I'd buy a condom.' Underneath, the copy reads: 'Introducing Mentor Contraceptives. The Smart New Way to Protect Yourself.' At the bottom of the page appears a photograph of a packet of Mentor condoms, and underneath the caption 'Smart Sex in the 80's'. So effective was this campaign, along with others, in shifting the audience away from heterosexual men's magazines such as *Playboy* to a heterosexual women's market that unmarried women were found in a study to have used twice as many condoms in 1987 as they did in 1982 (cited in Gamson, 1990: 273). Framing the condom as a 'beauty aid, a personal hygiene item, a public service' (Gamson, 1990: 274) involved disassociating it from its role as a contraceptive device. The disassociation of the condom from contraception and (hetero)sexual pleasure is crucial, according to Gamson, in breaking down the US media's opposition to condom advertising in newspapers and magazines, a strategy which proves more difficult to achieve with the major television networks.

The promotion of condoms to heterosexual women in the US is, however, met with resistance. An article in the magazine *Cosmopolitan* in January 1988 featured an interview with the physician Robert Gould who claimed that 'there is almost no danger of contracting AIDS through ordinary sexual intercourse' (Treichler, 1992: 22). Instead of reassuring millions of women readers about AIDS, the article had a negative impact in raising women's awareness about HIV and the need to protect themselves by practising safer sex. What is most startling about Gould's claims that 'penile penetration of a well-lubricated vagina – penetration that is not rough and does not cause lacerations' is safe, is that 'he also means *unprotected* heterosexual penile-vaginal intercourse *with an infected man*' (Treichler, 1992: 22–23). In the article Gould also claims that the high incidence of heterosexual AIDS in Africa is caused by the way 'many men in Africa take their women in a brutal way, so that some heterosexual activity regarded as normal by them would be closer to rape by our standards' (Treichler, 1992: 23). In response to this article the AIDS activist organisation ACT UP protested at the office of *Cosmopolitan* and distributed flyers challenging Gould's racist comments and the view that American women were not infected with HIV or dying of AIDS. So effective was this action that according to Treichler it 'marked a significant step forward in understanding the realities of the AIDS epidemic for women and in challenging prevailing representations' (1992: 23).

AIDS and race

Whilst the majority of women with HIV and AIDS in the US are black and Hispanic, the mainstream media in the 1980s 'had been silent on the rise of AIDS in the black and Hispanic communities' (Hammonds, 1986: 34). The phenomenon of heterosexuals with AIDS or heterosexual AIDS as reported in the mainstream media in the late 1980s is based on the assumption that these 'heterosexuals are white – read as white, middle-class, non-drug using, sexually-active people' even though there are few cases of AIDS among this group (Hammonds, 1986: 34). The startling picture of the missing story of AIDS and African Americans is well illustrated in Cohen's extensive study of the mainstream media's coverage of AIDS. Examining the *New York Times* from 1981 to 1993, Cohen finds that whilst the *Times* printed 4,671 stories on the AIDS epidemic, only 231, or 5 per cent, of those stories had African Americans as their focus (1999: 160). Of those stories which featured African Americans the majority were not related to the manifestation of the epidemic in black communities, but concerned black celebrities with AIDS (1999: 161). Cohen also finds a neglect of African American communities in the coverage of AIDS in network television evening news stories. The problem with this neglect is the possibility that 'people of color interpreted this absence as a signal that the AIDS epidemic was not about them or their community' (1999: 181). Cohen's concerns are confirmed by Sobo's (1995) research on AIDS-risk denial amongst disadvantaged women. In her anthropological study of African American heterosexual women from Cleveland (conducted between 1991 and 1993) she found that the majority of these women usually chose to forgo condoms. They did so because they did not think that they would catch AIDS. 'Most participants believed, as do most U.S. adults, that they were simply not at risk for AIDS' (Sobo, 1995: 2–3).

When African Americans are mentioned in mainstream press reports of AIDS they tend to be described in racist terms. Discussing an article which appeared in the Febuary 1987 issue of *Atlantic Monthly*, Hammonds draws attention to the main focus of the article – 'the risk of AIDS to white heterosexuals and the need for them to face their fears of AIDS so they can effectively change their behaviour' (1986: 35). In the same article it is debated 'whether certain "groups" of people have the same ability to exercise control over their sexual behaviour and drives as "normal" heterosexuals do' (Hammonds, 1986: 35). According to Hammonds, the categorisation of certain 'groups' as distinct from normal white heterosexuality, resonates with nineteenth-century views of syphilis. 'One of the primary differences that separated the races was that blacks were more flagrant and loose in their sexual behaviour – behaviours they could not control' (Hammonds, 1986: 31).

In the late twentieth century I want to suggest that this categorisation of African American sexuality as distinct from white heterosexuality concerns *the object of the condom*. In Chapter 2 I showed how the inscription of the African American body as sexually out of control is produced by a *cultural imaginary of condom use*. Drawing on the work of Patton, I pointed out this was particularly evident in relation to 'youth of color' who are represented as 'walking time bombs of violence and AIDS' (Patton, 1995a: 339). The ability to *choose* safer sex is not seen as a capacity of young black male bodies who are positioned as out of control, less vulnerable and innocent and therefore *in need of protection*. Such a representation of African Americans is not entirely new. According to Ferguson (2000: 423), in the twentieth century the 'construction of African-American sexuality as wild, unstable ... locates African-American sexuality within the irrational and therefore outside the bounds of citizenship machinery'. In the context of AIDS I want to stress that the construction of African American sexuality as wild and irrational concerns the perceived inability of black youth to be reflexive about the risk of HIV and choose safer sex. Whilst media representations of AIDS and safer sex education policies fix young black bodies as 'deviant' and 'premodern' (Patton, 1995a: 351) – and therefore 'needing to know about safer sex' (Patton 1995a: 339) – they simultaneously constitute the white adolescent body as capable of choice and the management of sexual risk and safety. In this way the condom produces racialised differences. It both becomes an extension of white middle-class future-oriented (hetero)sexual adolescent subjects and positions the body of the black youth as having no future.

The condom and the nation

To address this issue further let's return to the Australian Grim Reaper advertisement. What is interesting to note in regard to the discourse of safer (hetero)sex in the advertisement is the way it is framed in nationalist sentiments – 'AIDS could kill more Australians than World War II'. And in addition, the way in which the message of condom use – addressed to 'you' who 'can help stop AIDS' – 'If you have sex, have just one safe sex partner, or always use condoms – always!' is delivered to the audience in a *language of choice to care for yourself and the nation.*

In her analysis of contemporary advertisements and the discourse of choice Cronin has argued that in consuming such advertisements the self should not be understood as a preconstituted category but as 'performatively produced through the very discourse of choice' (Cronin, 2000a: 279). Moreover, Cronin shows how it is young male consumers who are predominantly addressed in terms of choice. Contemporary advertisements which address young men as self-reflexive provide a privileged position from which male consumers can 'contest cultural rights and belongings' (Cronin, 2000b: 8). If we consider the way in which the image of danger posed by the Grim Reaper who 'rages, chooses and kills' 'ordinary' (Lupton 1991, 1993) 'white, respectable and healthy "middle Australia[ns]"' (Tulloch and Lupton, 1997: 40) including a vulnerable housewife, baby, little girl and footballer is delivered to the audience in a language of *choice* to protect the self and the nation from AIDS (by *using a condom*) then the condom may be understood to concern the making of self-reflexive Australian male citizens.

The 'positioning of the "family" and "innocents" (particularly the mother, little girl and babe-in-arms) as "at risk"' (Lupton and Tulloch, 1997: 41) in the close-up shot of a 'stereotypical' group of victimised ten pin bowling pins, who are finally destroyed by the bowling balls of the Grim Reaper, may also be read as suggesting that the image of Grim Reaper threatening 'ordinary' Australians secures a *heterosexual self-identity*. As Fuss (1991) explains:

> The language and law that regulates the establishment of heterosexuality as both an identity and an institution, both a practice and a system, is the language and law of defence and protection: heterosexuality secures its self-identity and shores up its ontological boundaries by protecting itself from what it sees as the continual predatory encroachments of its contaminated other, homosexuality.
> (Fuss, 1991: 2)

Lupton's reading of the Grim Reaper advertisement as blurring the distinction between gay and straight sexual identities in relation to HIV/AIDS risk may thus be understood to normalise heterosexuality and overlook the way in which the figure of the Grim Reaper establishes heterosexuality as an identity and an institution through the language and law of defence and protection.

In an evocative account of heterosexuality and the public sphere Berlant argues that the 'state of sexual emergency' generated by the AIDS crisis is fuelled by a 'conservative rage against non-heteronormative forms of sexual activity and identity' (1997: 17). In Berlant's analysis the threat of AIDS to heterosexuality concerns the fact that 'heterosexual life no longer seems the only mentionable one' (1997: 17). Berlant suggests this is the case because the medical and political crisis created by AIDS increased public consciousness of gay people and increased public interest in lesbian and queer culture and non-reproductive heterosexual activity. The culture of AIDS in the 1980s thus 'made it *impossible* to draw an absolute public boundary between U.S. citizens and gay people' (1997: 17, my emphasis). In response to this breakdown of sexual boundaries she finds 'a virulent from of revitalised *national heterosexuality ... a form that is complexly white and middle class*' (1997: 19, my emphasis). What constitutes this national heterosexuality is a public sphere redefined in terms of intimacy with citizenship measured by 'personal acts and values, especially acts originating or directed toward the family sphere' (Berlant, 1997: 5). Even private acts like sex are now 'having to bear the burden of defining proper citizenship' (1997: 5). Since the mid-1980s ideas of nationality and sexuality in the public sphere have become so intertwined that according to Berlant the intimate – especially personal acts and identities – now defines what it is to be national, what is required to preserve the nation as well as protect the national future, a future that Berlant (1997: 21) argues is waged on behalf of the figure of the youth or child. What is especially pertinent to Berlant's account of the cultural dominance of heterosexuality and the privatisation and heterosexualisation of the public sphere is the changing role of the culture industries and popular culture in generating a shift in the definition of citizenship and national identity away from issues concerned with the state to those of intimacy and private sex acts. 'There is a vast culture industry generating text and law on behalf of heterosexuality's preservation and extension into resistant or unincorporated domains of identification and fantasy' (Berlant, 1997: 16).

Berlant's account of national heterosexuality has much to offer for an analysis of the Grim Reaper campaign. First and foremost, the television advertisement is an example of the mass media's capacity to produce a scene of national identification via the iconic figure of the Grim Reaper. As mentioned previously audience research has consistently shown that the image of the Grim Reaper had a lasting impact in the minds of Australians. Second, this television advertisement brought nationality and sexuality together in the mass mediated public sphere by redefining national identity in terms of the private sex acts of Australian citizens.

The audio discourse 'if not stopped, [AIDS] could kill more Australians than World War II. But AIDS can be stopped, and you can help stop it. If you have sex, have just one safe sex partner, or always use condoms – always!' suggests that AIDS – like war – is constitutive of a national crisis, and the threat to the nation comes from sex itself. The positioning of 'you' the audience as having the ability to 'stop it' makes the intimate and personal lives of Australians come to bear the burden of protecting the nation and the nation's future. In this sense the act of monogamous heterosex (having one sexual partner) *or* safer sex (heterosex with condoms) are defined as practices of national heterosexuality. This contrasts with the US where Patton argues that 'safe sex is the civic obligation of the gay citizen' who alone must take active steps 'to avoid polluting the nation' (1998: 363). Moreover, in the Australian context the civic obligation of the heterosexual population to practice monogamy *or* safer sex is waged on behalf of the future citizen – the child and youth. The image of white, respectable and healthy 'middle-Australians' being killed by the Grim Reaper ends with the shot of a little girl crying in fear whilst being knocked over by a bowling ball, and finally a baby being knocked from its mother's arms as both are bowled over by the giant ball. Here the figures of the dead child and the baby represent the threat of AIDS as a threat to Australia's future generations, and especially its national future.

Safer sex and adolescence

Audience research found the advertisement to have a resonating effect on the Australian youth population particularly in terms of promoting condom use for future safer (hetero)sex practices. In Lupton and Tulloch's study of 1005 year twelve students from New South Wales, the researchers found: 'Quite remarkably, nearly all participants in all groups remembered the "Grim Reaper" advertisement, even though they were only about seven years old when it was shown for a brief period of only two weeks in April 1987' (Lupton and Tulloch, 1996: 36), and that 'male students compared with female students ... rated television more highly' as a source of AIDS information (Lupton and Tulloch, 1997: 536). In Tulloch's (1992) survey of nine hundred Sydney school students, the majority of these respondents who chose television as the 'most important source' of AIDS information, also nominated the Grim Reaper advertisement as the most effective television representation in relation to HIV/AIDS education (Tulloch, 1992: 14). 'When asked to nominate the best ways of encouraging young people to use condoms during sex', Lupton and Tulloch found that of those secondary school students who rated television most highly as a source of AIDS information, 'the most popular choice was "a TV ad campaign with shock-horror pictures"' (Lupton and Tulloch, 1996: 41). Tulloch (1992) and Lupton and Tulloch (1996) also found that the image of the Grim Reaper and the accompanying message 'have a regular partner or use a condom always' to be the *most* effective representation in terms of encouraging young men to use condoms in the future.

In conducting focus groups, surveys and semi-structured interviews with this adolescent sample Lupton and Tulloch attempted to measure the effectiveness of national television representations of AIDS such as the Grim Reaper advertisement in raising awareness of safer sex and condom. On face value these qualitative and quantitative studies indicate that the Grim Reaper campaign successfully delivered AIDS information to the general population and increased knowledge of condom use, especially for adolescent males. But whilst the views of young people point to a shift in the meaning of AIDS and the condom in the mid-1980s to concern heterosexuality, this is enacted not only by the representation of HIV/AIDS on national television but also by the audience studies themselves.

In Chapter 2 it was argued that qualitative research methods are involved in the making of a certain kind of adolescent subject. I suggested that this process is at play in social science research on young people and condom use in which adolescents are asked to talk about the condom and provide an account of their present and future safer sexual experiences. It was argued that the telling of safer sex stories by adolescents is a technique through which the adolescent perceives himself or herself as having a future-oriented (hetero)sexual identity. Whilst Lupton and Tulloch consider their research findings on the Grim Reaper to reveal the impact of AIDS media campaigns, their research questions on future condom use may similarly be understood to concern the making of a national (hetero)sexual identity. For instance, in their attempts to measure AIDS awareness there is a sense of rightness and normalcy embedded in the condom for the practice of safer (hetero)sex, a practice which is understood to protect Australia's future generations.

The condom and whiteness

Television audience studies also illustrate the extent to which the heteronormativity embedded in the condom is complexly white and middle-class. This is evident in Tulloch and Lupton's research findings on the Vox Pop condom advertisement which was broadcast on Australian national television in 1990. In an investigation of the campaigns effects on young people Tulloch and Lupton (1997) draw attention to a particular sequence in the advertisement whereby 'an Italian-Australian youth gives a hip-thrusting gesture as he shows the *condom* in his wallet and says carrying condoms with you is good' (Tulloch and Lupton, 1997: 151, my emphasis). Tulloch and Lupton found 'a number of responses about this character condemning his attitude towards sex' (almost entirely from the girls): '"has sex for fun, not caring", "acts like he uses girls for one thing only", "makes sex look dirty" and so on' (Tulloch and Lupton, 1997: 173). In addition, they found that 'many participants indicated that the "ethnic" or "Italian" or "European" or "foreigner" or "wog" as the character they most disliked' (Tulloch and Lupton, 1997: 152), 'with 25 per cent of responses of "the wog loves himself, thinks he's a stud" variety, plus 12 per cent said "he looks like a liar" or "didn't speak good English"' (Tulloch and Lupton, 1997: 173).

The description of the Italian-Australian male youth as the 'Other', 'wog' and 'foreigner' resonates with Ang's (1995: 69) discussion of how southern European immigrants to Australia (which included Italians and Greeks) in the postwar period were 'perceived as non-white, thus "black"!' The reading of the 'wog' in the 1990 Vox Pop audience study as 'has sex for fun, not caring', 'acts like he uses girls for one thing only', 'makes sex look dirty' also resonates with Braidotti's (1997: 135) account of attending a Melbourne high school in the 1970s. Braidotti draws attention to depictions of herself and other ethnic youth in a novel written by one of her teachers, Helen Garner: 'Take Angelo [a character in the novel] for instance, with his volatile and sympathetic face, "making violent rabbit-like fucking motions with his hips"'

(Braidotti, 1997: 135). Garner's emphasis on the body of 'Angelo' and in particular his sex drive resonates with the audience response to the Italian-Australian in the Vox Pop advertisement. According to Tulloch and Lupton the 'audience response to *visual gesture* helps construct the actor as other' (1997: 152). 'The reasons given concern his *body language*: 'he thought he was a stud', 'his actions of having sex were disgusting' (1997: 152).

What is also significant in this reading of the actor as Other is the *visibility of the condom* in the actor's wallet. The audience's response to the 'wog' in the Vox Pop study as 'not caring' and 'making sex look dirty' positions the ethnic male youth – with condom in his wallet – as not concerned about HIV and *safer* sex. These findings thus draw attention the racialising aspects of the condom. The comment of a young Australian aboriginal woman taken from a focus group of young people's views on condoms in the mid-1980s further illustrates this point. Her response to the discourse of safer sex, 'I think it's more of a white person's sort of awareness' (Chapman and Hodgson 1988), is suggestive of the ways in which AIDS awareness and the issues of self-responsibility and self-care associated with safer sex may be available only to certain youth, specifically white adolescents. Moreover, the comment 'I think it's more of a white person's sort of awareness' highlights the extent to which sexual knowledge about HIV and its prevention concerns the making of white reflexive adolescent subjects. The condom could thus be understood as having 'constitutive effects in making, bodies, worlds and selves' (Franklin, Lury and Stacey, 2000: 7) whilst at the same time it is 'manifest at the level of knowledge practices and the *production or recognition of difference*' (Franklin, Lury and Stacey, 2000: 5, my emphasis).

AIDS research and the creation of difference

To address the issue of knowledge practices and the production and recognition of difference in relation to safer sex let's turn to some empirical studies. Focusing on the research of Wight (1999) on white working-class male youth from Glasgow and Rosenthal *et al.* on ethnic youth from Melbourne (Rosenthal, Moore and Brumen, 1990, Moore and Rosenthal 1992) I seek to highlight the assumptions of social researchers regarding difference and the consumption of safer sex information.

In the early 1990s Wight conducted a series of research projects in Glasgow on young heterosexual men and safer sex. Wight's focus was young men's sexual practices and their perception of HIV risk. In his research Wight 'explores how far an analysis of cultural factors is useful for making sense of data' (1999: 739). What is interesting to note in Wight's discussion of his empirical findings is the way he considers white working-class heterosexual male culture to have a negative impact on the ability of some men to respond to health campaigns promoting safer sex. Class differences are discussed in terms of who is (and who is not) capable of responding to the discourse of safer sex in media representations promoting condom use. Wight suggests that for the majority of unemployed, unskilled manual workers in his sample 'it is understandable that they *were unresponsive to public broadcasting of HIV education based on individual responsibility for one's health*' (Wight, 1999: 746, my emphasis).

Wight's analysis of working class masculinity – as unresponsive to media representations of the condom – contrasts with his analysis of middle-class men 'in higher education or professions' (Wight, 1999: 747) who are read as having the capacity to choose safer sex.

> Nearly all had practiced safe sex consistently with some, if not all of their partners *because of concerns about HIV*. There was evidence that several of them took *personal responsibility for their health and for practicing safer sex*, or were encouraged to do so by their parents. (Wight, 1999: 745, my emphases)

Whilst concerns about HIV may well involve issues of responsibility and care as Wight suggests, especially for this middle-class white male sample (assumptions I address in Chapter 7), what is most striking about Wight's analysis of safer sex is the assumption that social classes consume public health advertisements differently. What also stands out in Wight's discussion of cultural factors as either inhibiting or enabling safer sex awareness is the way the condom in the above discussion becomes an extension of a white middle-class identity. What I am seeking to draw attention to here is the way Wight differentiates between white middle-class heterosexual men as responsible for safer sex whilst positioning his working-class male respondents as unreflexive, that is not having the capacity to perform self-control, self-care, or indeed self-responsibility by *choosing to use a condom*. The assumption that young working-class heterosexual men are unable to read safer sex messages and change their sexual behaviour accordingly positions this group as unreflexive whilst at the same time suggesting that HIV/AIDS awareness is constitutive of a reflexive middle-class masculine identity (see Adkins, 2002 for a critical account of reflexivity).

To address further the impact of AIDS researchers in creating knowledge of difference let's consider an Australian study on adolescence and condom use. In the early 1990s Rosenthal, Moore and Brumen (1990) and Moore and Rosenthal (1992) conducted a series of empirical studies that investigated the differences in attitudes, behaviours and knowledge about HIV between Anglo-Celtic Australian adolescents and adolescents from ethnic groups, including Greek Australian, Italian Australian and Chinese Australian youth. In researching the relationship between adolescents and ethnic group differences Rosenthal, Moore and Brumen made the prediction 'based on the responses of older immigrants' that for non-Anglo-Celtics '*levels of knowledge will be lower and less positive social attitudes* will be evident than in the sample of Anglo-Australian adolescents' (1990: 222–223, my emphasis). They also argued that 'it is not unreasonable to expect that adolescents will be exposed to different responses to the AIDS threat as a function of their *cultural background*' (1990: 222, my emphasis). The researchers consider ethnicity to produce different kinds of effects in terms of the reception of safer sex messages by secondary school and university students. There is thus an assumption here that ethnicity or, as they conceive it, cultural background prevents the incorporation of media messages on the condom and safer sex into (hetero)sexual practices. What stands out in this account is the way cultural difference is measured in relation to the condom.

Not surprisingly, results from these studies revealed that there were *no* significant differences between non-Anglo and Anglo-Celtic Australian adolescents in terms of their responses to public health AIDS awareness campaigns. Whilst the researchers concluded that 'sexual contexts are highly complex, and vary almost as much between individuals as between groups' (Moore and Rosenthal 1992: 434), they nonetheless find this an interesting outcome of their research and go on to provide some rationale for doing further qualitative and quantitative research on perceived ethnic group differences in relation to AIDS education. Follow-up research, they argue, is necessary because their 'sample consisted of non-Anglo-Celtic adolescents who had *succeeded in the largely Anglo-Celtic education system*' (Rosenthal, Moore and Brumen, 1990: 236, my emphasis). But in claiming that the higher education system changes the behaviour of non-Anglo-Celtic adolescents the researchers assume that ethnicity is a fixed, stable identity which is incompatible with the development of a reflexive future-orientated adolescent (hetero)sexual subjectivity.

The cultural fixing of ethnic groups in health-related research has been widely critiqued. Fenton and Charsley (2000: 411), for instance argue:

> The supposed cultural attributes of ethnic populations are perhaps the most commonly advanced as implicated in the determination of health and illness. Frequently these are speculated upon or assumed rather than investigated and may include the following: family values, ... [and] attitudes to health care ... culture simply cannot be called upon in this way to 'explain' epidemiological patterns: when it is as several observers ... have pointed out, it pathologises minority groups.

Assumptions about culture are clearly at play in Rosenthal *et al.*'s research. The rationale for undertaking the initial research on non-Anglo-Celtic adolescents concerned the perceived inability of ethnic youth to respond to media campaigns promoting condom use because of their cultural background and family values. It was claimed that this group is culturally disadvantaged in its ability to educate itself about the risks of HIV and thus change their practices to include the use of condoms for the practice of safer (hetero)sex. Since the researchers measure ethnicity in terms of knowledge of safer sex, as opposed to say resisting or even interpreting the message of condom use differently, Rosenthal, Moore and Brumen (1990) and Moore and Rosenthal (1992) may therefore be understood to enact a form of cultural essentialism in their empirical study. Cultural essentialist accounts are enacted when 'culture is seen to be deployed as a fixed and fixing source of identity in ways which reproduce the previously naturalised hierarchies and exclusions of national citizenship and cross-national migration' (Lury, 2000: 158).

Given that Anglo-Celticness in Rosenthal *et al.*'s study is measured in terms of knowledge practices, safer sex campaigns such as the Grim Reaper advertisement may also be understood to concern the production of racialised differences. The comment 'I think it's more of a white person's sort of awareness' highlights the extent to which AIDS campaigns promoting HIV awareness and condom use constitute white subjects in contemporary multicultural Australia. If 'whiteness and Australianness can be accumulated (up to a certain point) and people can be said to be more or less White and Australian. How white they can be depends on the social attributes they possess' (Hage, 1998: 20), then the ability to possess the knowledge, skills and competencies to practise safer sex may indeed define a white Australian adolescent identity.

In drawing attention to AIDS representations of the mid-1980s this chapter has shown how the condom works in the interests of a national heterosexual culture whilst ignoring the needs of those most affected by HIV. Bringing together a range of mass media representations from the US, UK and Australia I have sought to highlight how the promotion of condom use in AIDS public health campaigns both constitutes a white middle-class adolescent identity and is constitutive of others who are deemed to be unaware, unknowing and uncaring of the consequences of unsafe sex. It was also shown that social researchers measuring AIDS awareness amongst adolescents have similarly produced social hierarchies and divisions in their interpretations of safer sex. The next chapter continues to examine media representations of AIDS and their constitutive effects. Shifting register to eroticised images of safer sex I address the impact of AIDS and safer sex discourse for understandings of the body, gender and sexual identity.

5
AIDS, pornography and the condom

In the previous chapters I discussed the impact of the mass media, school-based sex education and the social sciences in producing knowledge of the condom and (hetero)sexuality. In this chapter I consider the impact of social and cultural theory in the context of AIDS. I do so in relation to theories of pornography from the 1980s and 1990s. Addressing accounts of eroticised images of safer sex, this chapter aims to make explicit that, while there is much debate as to the effects of cultural representations and their relationship to identity construction, many cultural commentators share a number of theoretical assumptions regarding the body, gender and sexuality post-AIDS. This commonality concerns an assumption that the visual field, particularly vis-à-vis eroticised images of safer sex, works to break down and/or transgress a stable heterosexual masculine identity, to the extent that for many social and cultural theorists such images have been assumed to incite a crisis of the male body and a crisis of heterosexual masculinity.

In making this assumption explicit this chapter aims to problematise the 'male crisis' discourse. It does so by demonstrating that the general argument that the visual field in the context of AIDS has transformed sexual identities relies on a reading of images of bodies and body parts that are simply assumed to carry the marks of sexual difference. Two points are made regarding this theoretical assumption. First, I suggest that ironically such theoretical readings of the body and in particular the male body serve to stabilise the very gendered and sexed identities which the visual field is claimed to undo. Second, I suggest that this theoretical assumption (driven, as Kaite (1995) has made clear, by a semiotic analysis of representations) ignores the ways in which identity construction vis-à-vis the visual field takes place not simply with reference to images of bodies and body parts but with reference to cultural objects.

A number of analyses of pornography purposefully resist the dominant semiotic reading of the visual. This body of work is characterised by a refusal to get 'bogged-down' in engaging with the feminist debates on pornography and instead is concerned with the task of investigating the consumption of eroticised goods (see Juffer, 1998). What this body of literature suggests is that identity and identification can no longer simply be read off from eroticised representations but should be understood in terms of broader consumption practices.

Much of the discussion of pornography and consumption in the context of AIDS has indeed focused on the impact safer sex representations have had in constituting sexual communities, sexual vernaculars and to a large degree safer sex practices (Patton 1991a, 1991b, 1994, 1996). For instance, it has been argued that the consumption of safe sex materials by gay men has had important impacts on gay men's sexual culture (Patton 1991a, 1991b, 1996) and that the production and consumption of safe sex porn by lesbians constitutes a space from which to critique heteronormativity (Conway, 1996).

Whilst much of the literature on eroticised representations of condom use tends to assume that such representations affect non-heteronormative sexual others, in this chapter I argue that this reading of porn relies on the assumption of an already existing stable heterosexual masculine identity. The overall and very general aim of this chapter is to expose this assumption as well as the assumption of the transgressive potential of eroticised images, assumptions that operate across successive historical waves of analyses of porn. In making these assumptions explicit this chapter does not intend to prove that all previous accounts of pornography and or eroticised images are simply incorrect. Rather it aims to further develop an analysis of the history of the condom post-AIDS.

AIDS and pornography

In feminist analyses of pornography in the 1990s, particularly the writings post AIDS, the male body and the penis took centre stage. Feminist theorists such as Segal (1992, 1994, 1997), Williams (1990), Patton (1989), McClintock (1992), Bordo (1994, 1997) and Waldby (1995) were concerned with the differences between the representation of the naked male body and real men's bodies. In such analyses the phallus is figured in the context of the pornographic image itself, an image that contrasts with the real male body. This perceived difference between the 'representation' of the phallus and the 'real' non-phallic penis is associated with discourses on the male body in crisis. The discourse on male crisis is particularly evident in the context of AIDS discourse (Grosz, 1994: 198) and especially safe sex discourse (Singer, 1993: 84) which connect the penis to sickness and disease (see especially Segal, 1992: 82). According to Segal the advent of AIDS undermined the configuration of a corporeal phallic male body image (see also Patton 1994 and Wilton 1994, 1997). Indeed so strong is this threat that Segal states:

> Only in these two discourses [sexist pornographic and feminist anti-pornographic discourse] does the 'old male cock' continue to crow immune from more recent probings – especially in the 1980's and 1990's – that would connect the penis with every form of weakness from impotence to hysteria to sickness and disease. (Segal, 1992: 81–82)

In Segal's analysis, the representation of the penis as phallus 'the old male cock' is juxtaposed with the apparent phallic crisis currently experienced by (heterosexual) men, a crisis made worse by the condom in the discourse of safer sex, a discourse that is understood to increase the crisis in phallocentricm. This logic is illustrated particularly well in Segal's comments that many heterosexual men refuse to wear condoms because of 'men's need to prove their masculinity – their difference from women and from "poofters" – through a compulsive heterosexuality' (Segal, 1990: 165).

Such an argument suggests that the proliferation of safer sex discourse in the 1980s and 1990s concerns the 'dethroning of the phallus'. Yet is this the case? Kroker and Kroker (1991: xiv) argue that the discourse of the hysterical male concerns not so much the 'death of the privileged ideology of unitary male subject' but a newly emergent phallocentric order, whereby cultural power involves a return to the penis. This point is borne out particularly well if we consider the way in which feminist accounts of 'real' men's bodies in the context of AIDS – associated with sickness, disease and waste – produce a return to the penis. Thus whilst safer sex is understood to produce a crisis in masculinity and the death of a unitary male subject, this chapter examines how phallocentricism is reproduced in the context of theories of porn, AIDS and the condom. To begin I address the similarities in competing interpretations of pornography.

Feminism and pornography

In radical feminist analyses of the 1980s, cultural representations which are held to objectify the female body are deemed to be oppressive for women. Such images are perceived to produce the meaning of gender as sexualised power relations (MacKinnon, 1982, 1987a, 1987b; Dworkin, 1981; Jeffreys, 1990; Kappeller, 1986). This view is summed up well in the words of MacKinnon. (1987b: 148)

> Pornography institutionalizes the sexuality of male supremacy, which fuses the eroticization of dominance and submission with the social construction of male and female. Gender is sexual. Pornography constitutes the meaning of that sexuality. Men treat women as who they see women as being. Pornography constructs who that is. Men's power over women means that the way men see women defines who women can be. Pornography is that way.

By contrast feminist theorists of the 1990s took a more deconstructive position on porn. They suggested that radical feminist discourses on pornography in and of themselves define the meaning of gender as male-masculine-activity and female-feminine-passivity. Segal for instance argued:

> Sexual discourses and sexual iconography are seen to link dominant conceptions of female sexuality, and hence identity, with submission ... Yet, ironically, it is feminism itself (or strands of it), which is currently reaffirming the ties between heterosexuality and women's subordination. (Segal, 1994: xii)

> What we get from MacKinnon and Dworkin, both experts at the art of arousal and manipulation, is the discursive *mirroring* of the most disturbing codes and conventions of pornography itself. (Segal, 1998: 56 my emphasis)

Through a reading of the corporeal experience of heterosex, Segal attempts to get away from the 'mirroring' effect in such analyses of gender, a mirroring which she suggests problematically fixes the meaning of masculinity as male dominance and femininity as female submission. Segal's analysis is informed by the work of Brown (1995) who in her critique of radical feminist writings on pornography argues that MacKinnon's interpretation reflects 'rather than historically or analytically decodes' (Brown, 1995: 87) the representation of male dominance and female submission. According to Brown (1995: 87) 'MacKinnon's theory of gender unwittingly consolidates gender out of a symptom of a crisis of male dominance'.

In an attempt to liberate heterosexual women's corporeal experiences from 'sexually repressive feminist rhetoric' and oppressive pornographic representations (Segal, 1997: 80), Segal foregrounds 'the diversity and fluidities of heterosexual experiences and bodily contacts' (1997: 82). In particular, Segal (1997: 86) considers the materiality of the body in the act of sex as 'the most troubling of all social encounters' because 'it so easily *threatens* rather than confirms gender polarity'. For Segal (1997: 86) during sex 'the great dichotomies (activity/passivity, subject/object, heterosexual/homosexual) slide away'. Perhaps not surprisingly Segal's understanding of (hetero)sex as threatening rather than confirming gender polarity centres on the penis's performance, a performance which she argues undermines the rule of the phallus in straight male pornography, and the 'mirroring' of such male sexual subjectivity in radical feminist analyses of porn:

> The problem, of course, in admitting penile reference in conceptualizing the phallus is the changing condition of that particular bodily organ, between its transient firm and erect state and its more characteristic limp and flaccid (detumescent) one ... The phallus, in contrast, unaffected by time, context or desiring encounter, has no such temporal changeability, symbolizing (in its veiled way) the fantasy of the fullness and generative power of the always-erect penis. (Segal, 1994: 136)

By juxtaposing the phallus (an 'always erect-penis') with the vulnerable body part of the penis ('a limp and flaccid' 'bodily organ'), male corporeality is thus exposed as falling short of the representational phallus. Moreover, via her particular reading of

Butler's analysis of performativity as producing gender trouble and a 'subversion' of (hetero)sexuality (Segal, 1997: 88) Segal rethinks the idea of heterosexuality and male corporeality:

> whatever men's social power ... their actual sexual potency has always been precarious. Rather than endorsing the myths carried out by some of the most readily available in pornography ... we need to insist on the precariousness of bodily masculinity. (Segal, 1998: 59)

The corporeal logic at play in Segal's analysis of 'the precariousness of bodily masculinity' is also evident in the work of Bordo (1994: 265) who argues that 'the singular, constant, transcendent view of the phallus is continually challenged by its embodiment'. Indeed, according to Bordo 'the penis – insofar as it is capable of being soft as well as hard ... insofar as it is vulnerable, perishable body – haunts the phallus, threatens its undoing' (Bordo, 1994: 268).

These conceptualisations of the penis as undermining the symbolic phallus problematise radical feminist accounts of pornography as constitutive of gendered sexuality. In particular, Bordo's and Segal's analyses challenge the often-made claim that (dominant) male sexuality is constituted through the gendered act of looking at objectified female body parts and phallic male bodies. To this end there have been calls for a theoretical 'dephallicis[ation of] the hetero-sexual male body' since:

> full identification with this imago also requires a suppression of that in his body which confounds a phallic image. This suppression can be seen in the shame for men associated with 'impotence', having a soft penis or a penis which is 'too small'. (Waldby, 1995: 271)

At issue here is the physiology of the penis. On the one hand, male corporeality challenges the universal phallus. But on the other, the consumption of porn is understood to sustain an imaginary phallic corporeality. As Segal (1992: 69) puts it, 'through pornography ... delusions of phallic prowess [are] indulged, by imitations of the rock-hard, larger-than-life male organ'. And according to Bordo (1994: 267) 'only in pornography and homo-erotic representations do we see the phallus embodied in the erect penis':

> despite the 'pervasive presence of erections' in pornography, these

> are erections that are exposed precisely to be validated. Their validation – the transformation of embarrassed penis into proud phallus – is the point of pornography. (Bordo, 1994: 275)

What stands out in these analyses of porn is a conceptualisation of the phallus as defined by, and somewhat limited to, the image of the penis. Such a move is however called into question by Halberstam (1994), who argues that masculinity is not a property of men alone:

> The insistence ... that the penis alone signifies maleness, corresponds to a tendency within academic discussions of gender to continue to equate masculinity solely with men ... penises as well as masculinity become artificial and constructible when we challenge the naturalness of gender. (Halberstam, 1994: 214)

The conflation of the phallus with the penis in analyses of porn thus reinscribes a phallocentric logic in the sense that it prioritises the practice of seeing the difference, and returns us to a theory of the gaze whereby a masculine gender identity is presumed to concern an identification with a phallic male body image. But are the motivations of a contemporary masculine subject simply to validate a corporeal lack? Does this validation become greater for heterosexual men in the context of AIDS and safer sex? Does the condom challenge the naturalness of gender?

The gaze

Not all analyses of porn conflate the phallus with the penis. Williams (1990), for instance, in her account of hard-core porn points out that the performativity of the body part of the penis *within* the context of the photographic shot is 'an elaborately engineered and choreographed *show* enacted by professional performers for a camera' (1990: 147). According to Williams the symbolic status of the phallus is undermined by its performativity *as the phallus*. It is therefore 'simply not possible to regard a represented penis per se as a literal instance of male domination' (Williams, 1990: 268). Nor is it possible to interpret the consumption of the penis in porn as motivated by the viewing subject's desire for phallic reassurance, since the gaze is not sexed but transtextual. In other words, anybody can identify with the phallus in pornography. As Patton puts it:

we are sometimes voyeurs watching the action and sometimes in the eyeline of the male subject. But by the time of the come shot, the viewer is tightly positioned as the person who owns the penis. Even though not everyone in this culture has a penis, the cinematic conventions which position the viewer as the person coming are fairly seamless and it is quite easy to imagine that this is your penis, regardless of your anatomical configuration. (Patton, 1989: 105)

The act of looking at close up images of the penis-phallus is thus not restricted to a male audience. Thought of in this way the relationship between the representation of the phallus and the gaze, especially in the image of the come shot, can be understood to work against normative constructions of sexual difference, gender identity and sexuality.

Patton's reading of pornography as transtextual further undermines radical feminist analyses of the gaze whereby the act of looking at bodies and body parts is considered to be a dominant male activity that subsequently produces male sexual agency and female sexual insubordination. Indeed, Patton's (1996: 142) reading of pornography and the gaze as producing a 'range of positions in a variety of social spaces that create for each person a set of interpretative strategies' suggests that radical feminist analyses of porn which point to cultural representations as constructing fixed gendered subjectivities are misguided in their interpretation of the visual. Patton (1991a) draws attention to the way in which the pornographic imagination involves not so much a viewing male subject who interprets visual images as real events and then imitates these representations. 'Porn is not re-enacted but mimicked, subverted; it is not a manual but a site of memory, a repository of the phantasmagoric history of the body defying convention' (Patton, 1991a: 377). Patton's reading of porn also problematises Mulvey's (1990) influential thesis on the male gaze in relation to film. Specifically, Patton's point that the pleasure in consuming porn is not dependent on one's 'anatomical configuration' is a departure from Mulvey's thesis that 'the main male protagonist projects *his* look onto that of *his* like' (1990: 33–34, my emphasis).

Interpretations of the gaze as defined by one's anatomical configuration are further called into question by queer readings of porn which illustrate how visual practices may also cut across one's sexuality and race (see Fung, 1991: 154), and thus deontologise normative understandings of identification. But this is not to suggest that images of the body simply transgress sexed, gendered and racialised differences. In McClintock's (1992) account of straight porn she suggests that the image of phallic bodily fluids concerns not so much the undoing but the *making* of sexual difference. For McClintock (1992: 124) 'the cum shot restores gender decorum: the cum on the women's body marks her as separate, different'. In this reading of porn the image of phallic body fluids (on 'her' body parts) is understood as constituting and not simply transgressing the configuration of gender. But this realisation is not dependent on the expectation of seeing the difference in this way. In Dyer's (1982, 1985) analysis of porn, for instance, he argues that sexual difference is in no way compromised by the absence of women's bodies and body parts. Instead the representation of the penis and body fluids in the 'cum shot' constitutes a cultural imaginary of phallic male sexuality *without* the representation of women. Similarly Lehman (1993) stresses the expectation of seeing the penis as phallus in porn when he argues that 'large penises in pornography are also part of the need to make the "truth" of male sexuality visible and to affirm the serious visual drama of sexual difference that revolves around the penis as phallus' (1993: 155). What is thus highlighted in these accounts of porn and sexual difference is the visibility of the penis.

The male body

What I want to draw attention to here, in these rather disparate, contrasting and in many ways oppositional theoretical readings of porn, is the way radical feminist, post-structural feminist, queer theorists and gay film theorists tend to rely on and produce an account of the male body, and in particular the body part of the penis as phallic. This is especially the case in accounts of the male body in the context of AIDS. In claiming that in the era of AIDS heterosexual male bodies are 'all too readily exposed as fragile and destructible' (Segal, 1992: 83), an association is made between the penis and penile bodily fluids with disease, destruction, fragility and death. In so doing a comparison is made between the penis and the phallus. Thus in Segal's attempt to '*dethrone* the phallus through focusing on the penis' (Segal, 1992:

84) and the 'precariousness of bodily masculinity' she conflates phallic sexuality with a corporeal male body and in particular the body part of the penis. So whilst the equation of the penis with the phallus is considered by Segal amongst others (see Bordo, 1994; Waldby, 1995) to be naturally 'dethroned' through the performance of the real penis outside of the pornographic text, this undoing of gender also puts in place rather than straightforwardly challenges the ontology of the penis-phallus. In other words, accounts of male trouble which point to the body part of the penis as constituting a crisis for heterosexual men overlook the way in which such references to real male bodies restabilise gender, a stabilisation which occurs through theoretical re-evaluations of the male body in crisis.

In Wilton's (1994, 1996) analysis of porn and safer sex she too argues that the condom constitutes a threat to heterosexual men's masculine self-image and self-identity. According to Wilton condom use is 'feminizing' and 'intolerable within the terms of masculinity' (Wilton 1997: 34), 'constitut[ing] a tacit threat to heterosexual identity as "real" man' (Wilton 1997: 74). For Wilton the embodied practice of unsafe sex (without condoms) reproduces dominant heterosexual masculinity. Eroticised representations of the condom are considered to do little to encourage condom use since they fail to challenge the unequal power relations embodied in the practice of heterosex. 'The task of "eroticising safer sex" is just not that simple, nor is it one we should undertake without recognising our responsibility to challenge, rather than to collude with, the unequal social relations of power which are implicit in every sexual act, every sexualised text or image, and which act so powerfully to impede the practice of safer sex' (Wilton, 1994: 91). Whilst Wilton's position on porn is in many ways a departure from the views of Patton, Segal, Bordo and others, in the sense that Wilton perceives the visual to *maintain and reproduce* a phallic male subject and dominant male heterosexuality, Wilton similarly foregrounds male corporeality in her account of the eroticisation of safer sex.

According to Watney (1991, 1994) the negative response by radical feminists to safe sex porn activists (for promoting gendered heterosexuality) resembles local government sex education policies in Britain which banned the 'promotion' of homosexuality in the classroom. In the case of the Thatcher government's Clause 28 legislation, talk of lesbians, gays and safer sex in the classroom is seen to promote non-normative sexualities. In the case of the radical feminist critiques of porn, eroticised representations of safer sex are considered to reproduce dominant male heterosexuality and female sexual insubordination. Watney makes some interesting parallels here between feminist theories of porn of the 1980s and the British policy on sex education. What is evident in both instances, he argues, is the perceived role culture plays in the construction of sexual identities. According to Watney a negative response to eroticised safer sex images *'binds a theory of the formation of sexual identity with a theory of representations'* (1991: 391, my emphasis). Watney is critical of such views since a representational theory of sexual identity formation works against much-needed safe sex education. According to Watney the absence of positive pro-sex condom representations increases the transmission of HIV and also AIDS-related homophobia. 'Whilst individuals are vulnerable to HIV infection, the entire reproductive machinery of gay subjectivity is also vulnerable to the ideological fall-out of the representational crisis triggered by the virus' (Watney, 1989: 18). Radical feminist theories on pornography, particularly those in favour of its regulation and censorship, are seen as contributing to this desexualisation of gay culture and threatening gay subjectivity.

In making the argument that the representational crisis around AIDS throughout the 1980s amounts to the invisibility of positive gay subjects and a framing of gay sexuality as 'Other', Watney too produces a theory of representation which is linked with the formation sexual identity. More specifically, in his discussion of how the regulation of safe sex representations in the 1980s concerned a broader fear of homosexuality, Watney produces a theory of representation that is linked to the formation of heterosexuality. For instance, in arguing that 'the discourse on promotion therefore aims to saturate the image of the "homosexual" with the traditional connotations of depraved sexual acts, and to prevent cultural acceptability of gay identity, and sexual diversity rooted in the principle of sexual choice' (Watney, 1991: 400), Watney links the visual field in the context of AIDS promotion to the constitution of *sexual others* and in particular the figuring of gay as Other, a figuring which concerns the *stabilisa-*

tion of heterosexuality. What I want to address in the remainder of this chapter is the role of the condom in the stabilisation of heterosexuality.

Objects of knowledge

An analysis of objects is not lost in Kaite's (1995) discussion of pornography and difference. He argues that in pornography the female body 'is constructed through its discursive arrangement' (1995: 37), that is through objects that adorn the body. Kaite's reading of porn as 'as a discourse on sexuality that constitutes the body' (1995: 37) contrasts with Wilton's (1994, 1996) and Coward's (1982, 1984) definitions of porn in which the meanings of representations are understood to concern the objectification of 'women's' bodies and body parts as sexually available for the male gaze. However, as Kaite points out:

> this is to accept the 'woman as sign hypothesis', i.e., that representations of 'woman' are anchored around sexual difference, immediately recognizable and centred on the configurations of the body. But how do we know what we are looking at is a 'woman'? (1995: 13)

Kaite suggests that what is at issue in the pornographic text is not so much a sexualised female body and consuming male gaze but the way in which desire is produced through the visual construction of the body as sexed. Or, as Kaite (1995: 119) puts it, how 'the sexual fetish may in fact serve to sexualize the person'. Thus, in Kaite's analysis, the construction of sexuality in the pornographic text concerns the cultural object(s) which are mapped on to the body. For instance, he highlights how 'the artifacts adorning the body are as important as the bodily display itself' (Kaite, 1995: 39). In this way, the sexual differentiation of bodies is produced through the pornographic display of objects on the body. 'Sexual difference is a strategic deployment of signs' (Kaite, 1995: vii). 'This is the pornographic specular technique: desire on the surface of the body, not in it' (Kaite, 1995: 55). An analysis of pornography as constituting desire 'on the surface of the body' suggests that the terms of debate for analysing the effects of the eroticisation of the condom may be problematic. In particular, Kaite's understanding of pornography and sexual difference departs from feminist theories of representation which interpret the image of women's 'essential' body parts as either oppressive for women or misrepresentative of 'real' women's autonomous sexual desires and 'real' men's corporeal experiences.

In her study of women's domestic consumption of erotica and porn, Juffer (1998) shifts her focus away from what she perceives to be this dominant oppressive and/or utopic feminist framework for interpreting porn. She argues that such a shift is warranted since feminist interpretations of porn as either oppressive or transgressive are rhetorical in the sense that they then require further academic intervention:

> The problem with this emphasis on the violation of norms, or transgression, is not with transgression itself; rather it is that transgression seemingly exists in the aesthetic form itself and awaits the critic, who will make the *transgressive meaning* available for (appropriately trained) readers. (Juffer, 1998: 19, my emphasis)

For Juffer, claims involving the visual as a site of transgression concern not so much the popular text and the audience, but rather the academic field and feminist readings of porn. Juffer makes this point on the basis that existing feminist analyses of sexuality do not, in her view, address the issue of consumption practices and questions of identity formation but rely instead on interpretations of pornographic texts as either constructing or deconstructing women as social victims or liberated sexual agents. In contrast to these existing accounts Juffer addresses erotic 'texts as themselves sites where notions of home and sexuality are produced' (Juffer, 1998: 23) '*within* the routines of everyday life' (Juffer, 1998: 31). Juffer is primarily concerned with the way women's sexuality is constituted through and by the consumption of domesticated objects such as the vibrator and lingerie catalogues, and other commodities which she suggests are 'defined not by a set of internal properties, but rather by the nature of the exchange process' (Juffer, 1998: 25). In Juffer's analysis, porn and everyday life are not in opposition to each other, or indeed socially structuring or deconstructing of gender, as suggested in earlier feminist accounts of straight (male) porn.

Juffer's approach opens up porn and everyday life as a site where notions of sexuality may currently be constituted. Porn is defined as an empirical phenomenon, one that requires an investigation of the sociality of consuming porn in mundane domestic contexts. Whilst Juffer's methodology has obvious purchase (especially for understandings of female sexual pleasure) I want to examine her claim that a theoretical intervention will only ever amount to a process of new knowledge claims, for and on behalf of the feminist critic, whilst the actual consumers of porn are neglected. In particular, I want to critically address the transgressive logic Juffer locates at the heart of existing theoretical accounts of porn. In so doing I want to suggest that to abandon a study of feminist texts themselves, as Juffer proposes, may be to foreclose a history of knowledge production in relation to sexuality.

The condom and (hetero)sexuality

So far in this chapter I have shown how the male body has been a site for knowledge claims about the visual and identity formation, especially in relation to heterosexuality in the context of AIDS. In this final section of the chapter I focus much more closely on theoretical analyses of the condom in pornography. In Kipnis's (1996) thesis on pornography she suggests that porn 'may indeed be the sexuality of consumer culture' (Kipnis, 1996: xii), 'a form of cultural expression' (Kipnis, 1996: viii) that tells us 'about our history as a culture and our own individual histories – our formations of selves' (Kipnis, 1996: 167). Moreover, and if, as Kipnis suggests, 'the materials that constitute pornography are this close to the fundamentals of selfhood' (Kipnis, 1996: 206), then eroticised representations of safer sex may concern not so much the undoing of the sexual subject but perhaps its very formation.

Findlay (1992) describes this phenomenon nicely through her reading of an advertisement in which there is a close-up shot of what appears to be an individually wrapped condom tightly tucked into the back pocket of a pair of 501 Levis jeans. Within this particular image of safer sex Findlay considers the image of the condom as producing an eroticisation of (gay) safer sex to occur *without* the display of a sexualised male body or the body part of the penis. As Findlay puts it:

> In the case of the condom the idea is to swerve the sexual drive away from direct genital contact and onto an object used to cover the

penis. It tells the viewer that the condom in your back pocket is sexy. It tells you that the condom can be a fetish ... and eroticises everything about the man's body except his penis. (Findlay, 1992: 575)

What constitutes sexual desire and sexual identity and identification in the context of AIDS is not the representation of bodies and body parts but rather the condom itself. As Singer (1993) explains:

In both advertising and pornography, the goal is to incite arousal and satisfaction serially, that is to displace erotic investment on to other commodities, other items within the genre ... In this sense, then, pornography is not the discourse by which one body is represented to another body: it is a phenomenon of literacy, addressed to a reader of signs. Advertising is the mechanism for mobilizing this transferential logic in the direction of particular commodities. In pornography, the commodity is a sexual semiotic, that is a phenomena of sex without bodies. (Singer, 1993: 37–38)

In this sense, it would appear that the condom in the era of AIDS has externalised sexuality and sexual desire.

Whilst the impulse has been to suggest that the eroticisation of the condom concerns gay male culture, Conway (1996) in her analysis of the dildo and lesbian sex practices in the porno *Safe Is Desire* 1992 makes reference to the condom as constituting and constitutive of both gay and lesbian sexual desire:

Dionne and Allie's first date is cut short by the problem of unsafe sex, when Allie's gay neighbour opens his door on the kissing couple. He pleads Allie for a condom, which she produces from a special holder in her purse ... The favour is reciprocated when Dionne is handed a condom by the gay-signified man in the street. In these two scenes, apparently gay/queer men and women facilitate rather than compete against each other's sexual pleasure. (Conway, 1996: 138)

According to Conway this representation of safer sex and especially the dildo with condom destabilises, challenges and transforms ideas of the natural, the phallus and the embodied human subject. This takes place through 'strategies of inhabitation' (Conway, 1996: 149), strategies which involve lesbian actors taking up the dildo (with condom). The dildo and the condom thus challenge the conflation of the penis with the phallus since taking it up (and putting it on) is determined not so much by bodily masculinity but 'when the lesbian decides to deploy that erection' (Conway, 1996: 152).

In many ways Conway's analysis takes on board Butler's claim that the 'phallus is always plastic and transferable' (1992: 164). For Butler, the lesbian phallus not only works to challenge 'the stability of "masculine" and "feminine" morphologies' (1992: 160), it is also considered to 'resignify, unwittingly its own masculinist heterosexist privilege' (1992: 163). There are a couple of issues I want to raise here. First, I want to question whether Conway's analysis of the phallus is any different from those analyses I have presented so far in this chapter, especially feminist analyses of straight porn which have inadvertently rearticulated the phallus as a privileged signifier in their accounts of the male body in crisis, particularly in the context of AIDS. Is it simply the case that the lesbian phallus in producing a repetition of this signifier allows for 'the possibility of de-privileging that signifier' (Butler, 1992: 162)? And this leads to my second question. Does the plastic phallus (with condom) also work to resignify unwittingly a masculinist heterosexist privilege?

To answer these questions I want to consider the lesbian safer sex debates and draw attention to an underlying logic in two somewhat oppositional views on porn and condoms. In Conway's analysis of lesbian (safer sex) porn she suggests that the condom is constitutive of both lesbian sexual pleasure and a lesbian sexual identity. In other words, the condom is seen as transgressing heteronormativity. This view contrasts with that of G. Griffin (1998), who argues the object of the condom sits outside of everyday lesbian culture. The condom is '"not sexy" in two senses of that phrase: it has not – as yet – been conventionalized as part of erotic presentation' (1995: 151). Moreover, Jeffreys (1993) has argued that for lesbians the object of the condom does not constitute sexual desire, nor is it constitutive of sexual pleasure. Rather according to Jeffreys the condom concerns the 'imitation of gay male sexual practice' (1993: 138).

Even though Griffin's and Jeffreys's comments suggest that the condom is not (or not yet) part of lesbian erotic presentation I want to point out that they nonetheless bind a theory of the formation of lesbian sexual identity with a theory of safer sex representations. This is especially evident in Jeffreys's comment that lesbian safer sex porn concerns the representation of gay male sexuality and an imitation of gay male sexual practice. In analysing lesbian safer sex porn as imitative, as a copy of an original and more specifically as secondary to phallic male sexual practice, Jeffreys produces what Jagose (2002) describes as a cultural logic of sexual sequence, whereby female homosexuality is figured via its derivative nature. In other words, in her analysis of porn and safer sex, Jeffreys ironically produces a gendered account of sexuality she herself is so critical of. As Jagose explains:

> while identity formation based on homosexual desire between women is frequently represented in some belated or secondary relation to other forms of allegedly precedent sexual organisation, this is less an empirical fact concerning the date of their historical emergence than a constituent characterization of the masculinist and heteronormative representational strategies that secure the cultural definition of female homosexuality. (2002: 8)

For Jagose this relational configuration of lesbian sexuality, that is, as materialising by reference to male homosexuality and heterosexuality, operates to naturalise these sexual categories and sexual hierarchies. Attempts to address the question of lesbian (in)visibility in safer sex discourse thus run the risk of naturalising heterosexuality. Whilst these analyses suggest the condom *reproduces* or *challenges* and *deconstructs* the narrative conventions of porn which connect the phallus with male corporeality, such analyses are nonetheless characteristic of masculinist and heteronormative representational strategies which privilege male heterosexuality as precedent.

The logic of sexual sequence can also be seen to be at play in Conway's description of the porno *Safe As Desire*. According to Conway, the video produced an instructive representation of lesbian safer sex. As an educational porno for and by women *Safe As Desire* put lesbians at the centre of safer sex discourse and addressed the problem of lesbian invisibility and legitimacy in the era of AIDS. At the same time, the representation of the dildo with condom is understood to challenge the logic of the penis/phallus. But it is precisely this account of condoms as disturbing, *transgressing* and destabilising the phallus that Jagose's analysis calls into question. Specifically, in Conway's account of condoms as *transformative* of phallic (male) subjectivity and embodiment she produces a relational and derivative account of lesbian sexuality. At the heart of this transformational account of condoms and porn in the context of AIDS lies a theory of representation that naturalises the categories of heterosexuality and male gender identity as original, primary and authentic. What these safer sex debates, and the accounts of porn discussed throughout the chapter, highlight therefore is the significance of the condom for the constitution of sexual difference and heterosexual masculinity, issues which are explored in greater detail in the following chapter.

6
The condom, gender and sexual difference

The previous chapter showed how theories of porn have inadvertently naturalised the male body and heterosexuality as primary and authentic. This chapter shows how in the context of AIDS sociologists and social theorists have similarly produced a naturalisation of the male body and male heterosexuality in their interpretation of the condom in the context of AIDS.

Since the early 1990s a major concern in empirical studies and analyses of heterosex has been and continues to be why heterosexual men do not wear condoms. In the social sciences, and in particular the disciplines of sociology and psychology, heterosexual men's perceived reluctance to wear condoms is understood to be of significance since this reluctance is understood to have a negative effect in relation to public health campaigns which aim to reduce the heterosexual transmission of HIV/AIDS. Heterosexual men's apparent aversion to wearing condoms has led social researchers to ask why 'more people don't put one on' (Browne and Minichiello, 1994). Many commentators have suggested that the answer to this question lies in the way the practice of unsafe heterosex – without a condom – is a normative gendered act. Moreover, it is widely argued that the practice of unsafe heterosex embodies and is constitutive of hegemonic heterosexual masculinity. This view is summed up by Segal (1990: 165):

> many heterosexual men ... refuse to wear condoms ... Men's need to prove their masculinity – their difference from women and from 'poofters' – through a compulsive heterosexuality ... is in the context of AIDS, even more dangerous for women than it ever was before.

So strong is this understanding of unsafe sex as embodying normative heterosexual masculinity that it is commonly assumed that heterosexual men refuse to wear condoms. Even the increased visibility of the condom in popular safer sex campaigns is often understood not to change heterosexual men's resistance towards the condom.

In their attempts to explain this apparent disjuncture between the representation of the condom in safer sex campaigns and what is considered to be the dominant sexual practice of unsafe heterosex, many analysts turned to the idea of the male sex drive, and in particular Hollway's (1984) thesis on the discourse of the male sex drive. Drawing on this model of male (hetero)sexuality as an unstoppable force, feminists theorising safer sex have suggested that this model of male (hetero)sexuality has been reconstituted in the context of AIDS through the policy of targeting women in representations promoting condom use, such as the Australian 'If it's not on, it's not on' campaign. Moreover, the perceived need for heterosexual women to intervene and take responsibility to ensure 'it's on' is interpreted as reconstituting the ideology of male (hetero)sexuality as an uninterruptible, natural instinct. At the same time the cultural phenomena of the male sex drive is perceived to be disrupted by the discourse of safer (hetero)sex, in that women's responsibility for condom use is understood to challenge the normative and naturalised practice of (unsafe) spontaneous heterosex.

What stands out in such analyses of heterosexuality in the context of AIDS is that the discourse of the male sex drive is assumed, first, to be at issue, and, second, to be at issue only in the act of unsafe heterosex (without condoms). But in what follows I question the male sex drive – unsafe heterosex – thesis. By examining social research findings I will show that the male sex drive discourse concerns the act of safer heterosex *with* condoms. In so doing I argue that current understandings of the male sex drive as concerning the male body in the act of unsafe heterosex appear to take for granted the performativity of the condom and its impact in the making of sexed bodies and a heterosexual masculine gender identity. First, a brief history of the male sex drive.

Sexology and the male sex drive

According to Weeks (1985, 1986) the construction of sexuality by sexologists in the last decade of the nineteenth century was premised on the notion of a hydraulic sexual instinct. Through the use of metaphors such as 'overpowering forces, engulfing drives, gushing streams and uncontrollable spasms' (Weeks, 1986: 46), sexologists figured sexuality as an instinctual force. At the centre of this figuring of sexuality was the male body and male sexual practices. In the writing of sexologists instinctual metaphoric references were employed in relation to the body part of the penis. Thus it was the penis that came to be referenced as an unstoppable biological force. Moreover, this construction of the male sex drive as a capacity of the biological penis became normalised, since, as Weeks (1986: 46) notes, such discourses have proliferated and 'dominated the western discourse on sex'.

Via her reading of Foucault, Wood (1985) also understands the dominant depiction of sexuality as 'governed by biological processes' (Wood, 1985: 156) to constitute sexuality as an 'instinct' (Wood, 1985: 157). And for Wood what is key in the constitution of sexuality as an instinctual force is the discourse on heterosexual sex itself. As she points out:

> this sexual instinct is not, by and large, portrayed as purposeless energy, but as an instinct invested with a biologically ordained *aim* (intercourse) and *object* (usually a person of the opposite sex). (Wood, 1985: 156–157)

The discourse of (male) sexuality as a biological drive concerns 'how the instinct functions' in the context of (hetero)sexual sex (Wood, 1985: 157). Thus, as Bland (1996) points out, penetrative heterosexual sex becomes normalised and naturalised in the work of sexologists:

> In the early twentieth century and into the inter-war years, while sexologists ... *extended* the definition of the 'sexual', the definition of 'sex' itself was narrowed down into 'penetration' (and 'normal sex' into 'heterosexual penetration') ... Non-penetrative sexual activity was simply not 'real' sex. (Bland, 1996: 93)

In the late twentieth century the definition of normal sex as heterosexual penetration was in some ways challenged by the

AIDS discourse of safer (hetero)sex. Within this discourse the condom is widely considered to threaten heterosexual men's performance of real sex. As Coward (1987: 20) puts it, 'for men safer sex is seen as curtailment'. Similarly, Waldby *et al.* (1990: 181) argue that 'condoms compromise men's virility'. And according to Richardson (1990: 172) 'one reason men may be unwilling to alter their sexual behaviour is that they do not regard safer sex as sex. For them safer sex ... may seem a poor substitute for the real thing'. In short, condoms 'compromise manhood' (Kimmel with Levine, 1992: 321), by 'encourag[ing] men to stop having sex like men' (Kimmel, 1990: 107–108). The practice of penile–vaginal penetration *with condoms* is perceived to be especially problematic because 'it is in direct contradiction of the dominant social scripting of male sexuality, namely that it is uncontrollable or barely controllable force' (Wilton, 1997: 33). In these analyses the performance of hydraulic male (hetero)sexuality as an 'uncontrollable or barely controllable force' is understood to be at issue *only* in relation to the 'normal' practice of unsafe (hetero)sex, that is via the *absence* of condoms.

Unsafe sex and the male sex drive

Whilst the condom is understood to challenge the social scripting of male sexuality, the allocation of responsibility to women for the use of condoms in popular safer sex advertisements is understood to re-construct the male body as a natural force. As Scott (1987: 14) put it:

> in accepting uncritically that women are more responsible than men [for condoms], [the discourse on safer sex] fails to challenge male behavior and puts the burden of changing their acts and attitudes on to individual women. It takes as 'natural' men's resistance to self control.

Similarly, Richardson (1990: 172) argues

> despite exhortations to 'take responsibility for our own actions' underlying most prevention efforts there appears to be a tacit acceptance of the assumption that men are 'naturally' less able to exercise self-control when it comes to sex than women.

The message is that 'men have powerful sexual urges which they find difficult to control' (Richardson, 1993: 84). In discussing the 'If it's not on, it's not on' campaign Waldby (1996: 10) argues that 'heterosexual men remained unmarked, the unspecified force which women are asked to control, the force against which they need protection'.

At the same time the condom is read as problematising the hydraulic model of male (hetero)sexuality. According to Browne and Minichiello the slogan 'If it's not on, it's not on' 'not only implies that women must assert themselves – but also that traditionally accepted male sex needs/drives locate men in a compliant rather than active position in condom use' (1994: 243). This view is further evident in the work of Richardson, who argues that the construction of normative female sexuality as 'passive and male as 'active' ... [is] threatened by the allocation of responsibility for negotiating sexual practices to women and the demand they take active control over the sexual encounter' (1996: 174). Condom use is thus considered to challenge the social production of male sexuality as active as well as the construction of female sexuality as responsive to men's culturally constituted biological sexual instincts.

So prominent is this interpretation of the male sex drive in relation to the practice of heterosex *without* condoms that some sociologists have suggested that heterosexual women who insist on the use of condoms for the practice of heterosex threaten the construction of male heterosexuality. Wilton and Aggleton (1991: 155) for instance, argue:

> Heterosexual women who attempt to ensure their partners safety by suggesting the use of a condom ... introduce an element of *premeditation* into an act justified largely by its *spontaneity* ... and they ask their partner to behave with a responsibility which is simply dissonant with the construction of the male sex 'drive'. Furthermore, to purchase and carry condoms is, for a woman, to challenge the patriarchal definition of her sexuality as innately responsive to male initiative. (my emphases)

Similarly, Holland *et al.* (1991, 1998) and Thomson and Holland (1994) suggest:

> Condoms symbolise breaking the flow and destroying his passion. (1998: 37)

> When a young woman insists on the use of a condom for her own

The condom, gender and sexual difference 101

safety, she is going against the construction of sexual intercourse as a man's natural pleasure. (1991: 131)

Requesting or insisting on condom use in this context can be a potentially subversive demand. The spontaneity of passion can be undermined. (1994: 24)

The condom is thus understood to question and potentially subvert the social construction of men's 'natural' sex drive.

The practice of safer heterosex is seen to be especially problematic for adolescent males. For young men the performance of 'real' and 'natural' sex 'concerns technique' whereby the man is positioned as the 'initiator' and is expected to know 'how to go about it' (Crawford *et al.*, 1994: 581). And for Holland *et al.* (1996b) the achievement of such a sexual technique is understood to be particularly at issue during their *first* experience of heterosex:

First intercourse ... is part of a much more general, and less visible, process of induction into the dominance of masculine norms and meanings as 'natural' ... 'First sex' is the key act by which they become a man. (1996b: 145)

Significantly, this moment of dominance is achieved by a man losing his bodily control. (1996b: 150)

For a young man, achieving intercourse is an empowering moment of symbolic and physical importance, whereby through a physical performance, his identity as a man and, therefore, a competent sexual actor is confirmed. (1996b: 158)

The problem of safer sex according to Wilton (1997) is that the condom jeopardises the performance of natural heterosex and undermines the achievement of a heterosexual masculine identity:

If we consider condoms, it becomes obvious that for a man to use a condom while having sex with a woman is ideologically risky. He is putting his masculinity at risk by doing so because condom use is feminizing ... He is demonstrating a degree of control over his sexual behavior which is feminizing ... Safe or safer heterosex is ideologically intolerable within the terms of masculinity. (Wilton, 1997: 33–34)

Patton perceives the threat of the condom to the maintenance of a heterosexual masculine identity as so profound that she argues 'it seems baffling that ... the use of a condom ... is greeted by heterosexual men as if it were *tantamount to castration*'. (1994: 114, my emphasis)

In Jackson and Scott's (1997) sociological analysis of (hetero)sexuality they suggest the reason why men don't like condoms and women find it difficult to convince men to practice safer heterosex concerns broader social inequalities:

> getting men to use [condoms] was not so simple. Public discourse around safer sex in this period can be understood within a post-Fordist frame, with a focus on re-skilling and increased flexibility. Heavy male sex work, with the emphasis on performance, seemed to be of less value and female negotiating skills came to the fore. Meaningful negotiation, however, requires an equal starting point and *most health advice has ignored the inequalities within the gendered dynamics of heterosexuality* (Holland et al., 1990[c]) ... In the end, this public discussion has taken a form which offers minimal challenge to male sexuality. (Jackson and Scott, 1997: 564–565, my emphasis)

If the public discussion of condom use 'offers minimal challenge to male sexuality', since the discourse of safer sex which encourages women to negotiate condom use with men 'ignores the gendered dynamics of heterosexuality', then it would appear that heterosex without condoms is indeed a site of male power.

But whilst this analysis of the performance of 'heavy male sex work' (heterosex without condoms) suggests that the male sex drive concerns the *social* construction of gendered heterosexuality, Hollway's (1984) analysis calls into question such theoretical understandings of male sexuality. In particular, Hollway recognises that although these kinds of feminist interpretations of heterosexuality do indeed challenge the view of male sexuality as a 'natural' force, she also suggests that analyses of the male sex drive as concerning male (hetero)sexual power and female insubordination put in place another monolithic understanding of gender, one whereby a biological determinism is replaced by a social determinism. Hollway writes:

> True we have challenged men's 'natural sexual drive'. But we have replaced it with an idea of the power of the penis/phallus which, in another guise, grants men's sexuality a monolithic power over us. (Hollway, 1984: 63–64)

Hollway's (1984) concern is that contemporary feminist analyses of heterosexuality tend to map a universal model of gender relations on to the male body and especially the body part of the penis, a move which can indeed be seen in analyses of unsafe sex.

And to this we might add that since these accounts all rely on an understanding of men as reluctant to practise safer sex, they themselves produce – via a discussion of non condom use – the idea of hydraulic sexuality as concerning the body part of the penis. In other words, in analysing men's performances of unsafe heterosex as a gendered act these accounts not only put in place an understanding of the male sex drive as a fixed and inherent feature of male (hetero)sexuality, they also reproduce a definition of male sexuality as a naturally occurring biological instinct and the act of unsafe heterosex as a normal sexual practice. Thus, in their attempt to move beyond the 'repressive hypothesis' discussed by Foucault (1979), these analyses of safer sex ironically reproduce an account of male (hetero)sexuality as socially repressed and physically thwarted by the condom.

Moreover, in claiming that the public discussion of condom use 'offers minimal challenge to male sexuality' (Jackson and Scott, 1997: 565) these analyses do not address the discourse of safer sex. As Pringle (1992: 100) points out:

> Bodies have a meaning only to the extent that they are already situated within discourse ... contemporary theorists largely take for granted that we make sense of the world through discourse. Identities, whether as sexed, sexual or gendered are not pre-given. They have to be constructed, articulated and maintained: they do this using the discursive framework available to the time and culture.

In stressing that contemporary theorists of culture and the social must take into account 'the discursive framework available at the time' in order to understand the meaning of bodies and the constitution of identities, Pringle's approach contrasts with the analysis of heterosexuality and the male body offered by Jackson and Scott (1997). More specifically, in foregrounding the significance of the discursive framework for interpreting the meaning of bodies and the social construction of gender and heterosexuality, Pringle's account suggests that the performance of 'heavy male sex work' may be constituted in and by the very discourse of safer sex itself. Waldby (1996: 10) makes this point in her discussion of the 'If it's not on, it's not on' safer sex campaign when she suggests that 'heterosexual men remained unmarked, the unspecified force which women are asked to control'. Here the male sex drive is perceived to be constructed by the popular discourse of condom use which conveys the message that heterosexual men are reluctant to engage in the practice of safer (hetero)sex. Whilst Waldby's account of men's culturally constituted uncontrollable sexual urges appears to contrast with sociological analyses of the male sex drive which suggest that the performance of hydraulic sexuality concerns gender power relations, Waldby's account of the male sex drive is nonetheless somewhat similar to the sociological analyses in the sense that she also imagines hydraulic male sexuality to materialise only in the act of *unsafe sex* (heterosex with condoms).

Safer sex and the male sex drive

To examine whether this dominant interpretation of the male sex drive adequately gets to grips with heterosexual male condom use, particularly adolescent male condom use, I turn first to the findings of Holland *et al.* (1998). In their interviews with adolescent males and females in London and Manchester during the late 1980s and early 1990s Holland *et al.* find that the object of the condom is perceived to be somewhat incompatible with the 'the notion of men's natural and uncontrollable sexual drive which should not be interrupted or diverted' (1998: 36). What is most notable in their analysis of the male sex drive as taking place through the act of unsafe heterosex is that some of the interview material they draw on to highlight this process of interruption whereby 'condoms symbolise breaking the flow' (1998: 37) does not appear to demonstrate that the condom is experienced as necessarily interfering with the performance of a hydraulic male sex drive. For instance, the comments made by a male respondent –

> if you get that close to someone and you really fancy them badly and you get to that stage then you will probably end up having sex anyway, *with a condom or without*. There's that urge. (1998: 37, my emphasis)

– suggest that the experience of the 'urge' for this young heterosexual man was not limited to the practice of unsafe sex (without a condom), but also included the practice of safer sex (with a condom). The following comments taken from Holland *et al.*'s (1998) research findings further illustrate the ways in which safer sex and male (hetero)sexuality are not exclusively incompatible:

> Well condoms are a bit mechanical – not in themselves – it's just you put one on, then you have sex under cover, then you take it off again. (1998: 48)

> What I enjoyed about sex when we weren't using a condom was the fact that we could – like stop and start, we didn't have to – you know – do it ... You know we wouldn't have to do the whole thing because I'd had a condom on. (1998: 48)

The view of safer sex as 'mechanical' in that 'you put one on' and 'do it' 'the whole thing' indicates that having a 'condom on' was not experienced as 'interrupting the flow'. Moreover, these comments highlight the ways in which the condom itself produces hydraulic sexuality. These comments thus suggest that the condom does not so much interfere with the discourse of the male sex drive but could be understood via Butler's (1990) analysis of performativity as constitutive of a set of repeated acts that produce over time the appearance of a stable heterosexual male body as a natural instinctual and hydraulic force. Following Butler (1990) we could also analyse the male sex drive not as an essential internal force, nor as internal to the body, but produced as an effect of safer sex. What I'm arguing here is that gender is constituted by the performativity of the condom.

To examine this process further let's turn to research findings which show the practice of safer heterosex to be a common occurrence for male adolescents, particularly for first and initial acts of heterosex. In Lindsay *et al.*'s (1997) survey of 3500 Australian secondary students the use of condoms by fifteen- to sixteen-year-olds was found to be a normative act, with 74 per cent of the 171 male respondents surveyed in 1997 claiming that in the previous twelve months they 'always' used condoms when engaging in heterosex (Table A5, figure 5.4: 30). And in a smaller study of 244 young people aged between fifteen and eighteen in Victoria, Rosenthal *et al.* (1997) found high levels of condom use amongst high school students. In this study, 81 per cent of the 244 respondents claimed to have practised safer sex in their most recent sexual experience, with more young men (93 per cent) than young women (70 per cent) having used a condom during their most recent sexual experience. 'If a condom was used, it was more likely to be provided by the male than the female partner' (Rosenthal *et al*, 1997: 103). Similarly in Smith and Rosenthal (1997) Australian study of adolescent sexual practices during 'Schoolies Week' the majority of the male respondents expected to have sex while on their end-of-school holidays in Queensland (80 per cent), with 83 per cent expecting to use condoms and two-thirds of the young men actually practising safer sex with casual partners (Smith and Rosenthal, 1997: 175). Together these findings suggest the practice of safer sex may be quite normative for first and initial acts of heterosex. What I am seeking to highlight here is how the constitution of normative heterosexuality and its claim to naturalness concerns not so much young men's dis-identification with the condom in the discourse of safer sex, but an identification with 'it' – the condom itself.

And yet this particular interpretation of the condom is not considered in most accounts of heterosexuality and safer sex. In the Australian case, for instance, Waldby, Kippax and Crawford (1991: 39) are 'concerned with the absence of the heterosexual male body from government policies addressed to the prevention of HIV/AIDS transmission'. The absence of heterosexual male sexuality is noted in 'education campaigns [which] concern themselves with persuading women to protect themselves against the virus' (Waldby *et al.*, 1993a: 247). Waldby (1996: 10) foregrounds the 'If it's not on, it's not on' campaign as one which 'made quite explicit the assumption that women must act as the guardians of socially responsible sex, while the actual wearers of condoms are not addressed'.

> As the only group *exempt* from direct address by public health discourse they are freed from internalising the idea of their bodies as dangerous or infectious, relying instead on the willingness of heterosexual women to undertake such internalisations. Heterosexual men are thus allowed to maintain an (imaginary) position of the clean who are threatened from infection from below and elsewhere.
> (Waldby, 1996: 10)

In a discussion of British public health campaigns promoting safer heterosex Richardson (1990: 173) also finds 'men and their responsibility for the safety of sex are conspicuously absent'. 'The heterosexual male ... is largely invisible in AIDS discourse' (Richardson, 1996: 173). Wilton (1997: 94) too suggests that 'safer sex material targeted at heterosexual men is largely non-existent', and, like Richardson, uses the term 'invisible' (Wilton, 1996: 95) to describe the way in which she perceives heterosexual men not to be represented in AIDS discourse. Wilton's thesis on '*Nowhere Man*' (1997: 95) and Richardson's thesis on 'The disappearing heterosexual male' (1996: 167) may thus be read as quite similar in the sense that the heterosexual male body is understood to be 'invisible', 'absent' and 'non-existent' in the discourse of safer sex and HIV transmission.

Despite these similarities Wilton and Richardson perceive the absent and invisible male body in safer sex discourse as having rather dissimilar effects. Although Wilton and Richardson both consider 'the concentration on women as a source of HIV infection' (Richardson, 1996: 167) in AIDS discourse to 'construct a familiar model of women-as-risk to man' (Wilton, 1997: 69), the representation of heterosexual women as contaminating is read as having different implications for heterosexual masculinity in AIDS culture. Richardson, for instance, analyses the image of heterosexual women as a dangerous source of HIV infection as 'threaten[ing] the active/male, passive/female dichotomy' (Richardson, 1996: 174) and that 'such changes would represent a threat to male identity' (Richardson, 1990: 173) whilst Wilton considers this image to reproduce a dominant model of heterosexual masculinity:

> The body of safer-sex educational material developed to date, far from constituting any kind of radical 'new' discourse of the erotic, simply replicates the familiar constructions: ... heterosexual men represent the invisible 'norm' whose sexuality is so absolutely proper and right to resist problematization. (Wilton, 1996: 95)

AIDS and sexual difference

In contrast to these particular interpretations of the discourse of safer sex, Grosz argues that, in the context of AIDS, the condom concerns an inscription of sexual difference. In the text *Volatile Bodies*, she explains:

> It is women and what men consider to be their inherent capacity for contagion, their draining, demanding bodily processes that have figured so strongly in cultural representations, and that have emerged so clearly as a problem for social control. This has become alarmingly clear in contemporary AIDS discourse, where programs to halt the spread of the disease into the heterosexual community are aimed at women: women are, ironically, the ones urged to function as the guardians of the purity of sexual exchange. It is they who have been targeted by medical groups and community health centers as the site for the insistence on condom use. (Grosz, 1994: 197)

The targeting of women in contemporary AIDS discourse is thus considered to involve an association of women's bodies with 'their inherent capacity for contagion' and the simultaneous disassociation of the male body from such 'draining' and 'demanding bodily processes'.

It is the association of women's body parts with dangerous bodily fluids which is considered by Grosz to be key for understanding how sexual difference is produced in relation to AIDS discourse.

> The representation of the female body as an uncontainable flow, as seepage associated with what is unclean, coupled with the idea of female sexuality as vessel, as container, a home empty or lacking in itself but fillable from the outside, has enabled men to associate women with infection, disease, with the idea of a festering putrefaction, no longer contained simply in female genitals but at any or all points of the female body. (Grosz, 1994: 206)

In Waldby's (1996) thesis she too considers sexual difference to be produced through a cultural imaginary of women's bodies and body parts as fluid, as an 'infectious flow' (1996: 111) as opposed to solid. In the schemas of AIDS epidemiology such bodies:

> are considered to be implicated in the spread of infection because of their inherent *permeability*. (Waldby, 1996: 110, my emphasis)

> this lack of boundary is imagined not as a general formlessness but as a capacity for sexual receptivity, for the accommodation of phallic breach of their body boundaries. (Waldby, 1996: 105)

The imagined capacity of women's and gay men's body boundaries as 'permeable' and 'sexually receptive' produces a phallic male heterosexual subjectivity:

men are able to secure a self-image as stable, self enclosed and individuated, untroubled by fragmentation and confusion, only through projection of these fluid and cloacal qualities onto women. (Waldby, 1996: 77)

The association of women's bodies as 'a kind of fluid pathway' in AIDS epidemiology (1996: 106) is also considered by Waldby to be at issue in the discourse of safer sex. 'Women must be made responsible for safe sex practice because it is the cleanliness of their bodies which is at issue, not that of heterosexual men. *Women must be the guardians of safe sex because they are more implicated in infectious flow*' (1996: 111, my emphasis). Safer sex is thus understood to concern an inscription of the female body as fluid and the male body as phallic.

Waldby's account of safer sex and sexually difference is well supported by Roberts *et al.*'s (1996) research findings which reported that vaginal secretions were talked about by the male respondents in terms of 'disgust and a fear of contamination' whereas 'semen [was] fantasised as a symbol of masculine virility' (Roberts *et al.*, 1996: 114). According to Roberts *et al.* 'these attitudes towards semen are linked in a number of ways to the concept of imaginary bodies' (1996: 113), especially to the 'historical connection between women's genitals and dirt' (1996: 113–114). The configuration of 'men's bodies ... as phallic and impermeable' (Stephenson *et al.*, 2000: 111) and female corporeality as an 'infectious flow' (Waldby 1996: 106) is considered to be disrupted by the mixing of bodies in the (hetero)sexual encounter. Stephenson *et al.* (2000), for instance, following Roberts *et al.* and Waldby, suggest that untrustworthy women threaten masculine subjectivity. The development of a coherent sexed male body image is jeopardised by the potential for women's bodies to be permeable and sexually receptive to more than one male body. 'As long as she is faithful, he can penetrate her without coming into contact with other men's bodily fluids, and without the *fear of losing himself, losing his self-identity*' (Stephenson *et al.*, 2000: 112, my emphasis).

The (hetero)sexual encounter as a site of corporeal contestation?

The stability of a corporeal heterosexual masculine self-identity is also considered to be troubled and fragmented by the interaction of bodies, body parts and body fluids in the context of the (hetero)sexual encounter.

> If one aspect of the imaginary anatomy aspired to in the enactment of heterosexual masculinity involves representing the body as deployable at will and the self as self possessed, the arena of sex presents problems for the maintenance of this self-image. Sex (potentially) confronts its subjects with their debt to corporeality; the possibility of an external, rational relation of self to body is dissipated in the consequences of erotic pleasure. The imaginary anatomy of self-possession – the body as bounded, as amenable to control, as isomorphic with the subject's will – can be shattered in sexual relations, both because it disorganises the teleology of that anatomy, makes it (momentarily at least) 'polymorphous', and because it brings it into a confused relationship to the lover. (Waldby et al., 1991: 47–48)

An interpretation of sexual practices as transgressing the cultural imaginary of sexual difference suggests that what is 'shattered', 'disorganised' and 'confused' by the interaction of bodies and body parts in sexual relations is both a sexed male body image and a heterosexual masculine self-identity (see also Waldby et al., 1991; Waldby, 1995; Smart, 1996a, 1996b; Segal, 1997).

So strong is this interpretation of the space of the (hetero)sexual encounter and safer sex practice as outside of and moreover challenging a rational relation of self to body that Waldby (1995) perceives the corporeal experience as a possible site of subversion:

> A more sophisticated investigation of the bodily imagos of sexual difference and their implications for subjectivity must take into account a certain instability in what they mean and how they are lived out ... while an ideological reading would render sexual practice as the most pure point of the existence of the reductive bodily imagos I described above, it is possible to counter this along the lines that sexual practice, exactly because it involves erotic pleasure, is a potential site for their *subversion* and *reconfiguration* and for a correlative freeing up of their subjective implications. (Waldby, 1995: 270–271, my emphases)

In making the claim that the way in which bodies are 'lived out' in the site of the sexual 'must take into account a certain instability' of the 'bodily imagos of sexual difference', Waldby (1995) thus cautions against mapping social understandings of gender onto (hetero)sexual practices.

In Holland, Ramazanoglu, Sharpe and Thomson's (1994) study of AIDS and young heterosexual women in England, they too consider the sexed and gendered meaning of bodies and body parts to be (potentially) subverted through the interaction of bodies in the (hetero)sexual encounter. For Holland *et al.* (1994) the 'material' substance of women's bodies transgresses the 'social meaning' of the 'socially constructed body':

> The manifestation of material bodies is an intrusion into the romantic ideal of something that is smelly, hairy, *bloody; prone to spots, discharges, seepage, hormonal changes*; it is arousable, pleasurable, with erogenous zones ... Young people embarking on sexual encounters have to make decisions about ... how to manage *bodily fluids* and noises; ... what is deviant, dirty, unfeminine, unmasculine or otherwise not decent ... There is a tension here between the order of socially constituted, gendered identities, and the potential disorder of the uncontrollable body ... Sex connects bodies and this connection gives women an intimate space within which men's power can be subverted and resisted. (Holland *et al.*, 1994: 34, my emphasis)

What I want to draw attention to here is the ways in which the potential disorder of the uncontrollable body contrasts with Holland *et al.*'s research findings on the meaning of the lived body for young heterosexual men in the act of first heterosex. In some instances the sexual appears to be a space where a corporeal masculine self-identity is formed. That is, the sexual appears to be an important site for understanding the way in which the male body becomes sexed, and a masculine heterosexual self-identity is configured:

> First intercourse for young men was a challenge that could threaten their successful achievement of manhood. Their potency was at stake, they did not necessarily know what to do with their bodies, and there was a good deal of concern about doing it right. But in these positive accounts, the main point was to *do* it – a masculine performance in which they were the star player. (Holland *et al.*, 1996b: 147)

These findings indicate that the performance of the male body and especially the body part of the penis in the act of first heterosex are important for understanding 'manhood' and masculinity in AIDS culture.

These findings therefore call into question Segal's (1997: 86) claims that the performativity of body parts – 'including the most fragile of all appendages the penis' – 'wandering over, in and between the flesh of the other', necessarily breaks down the 'great dichotomies active/passive, heterosexual/homosexual'. As Holland et al. put it:

> For a young man, achieving intercourse is an empowering moment of symbolic and physical importance, whereby through a physical performance, his identity as a man, and therefore, a competent sexual actor is confirmed. (Holland et al., 1996b: 158)

This interpretation of the act of first heterosex as having material significance for young men echoes Connell's (1995: 56) view that 'the body ... is inescapable in the construction of masculinity'. But the comments of

> a young man [who] concludes that it is what is done with the penis that matters ... [and] the emerging consensus from young men that size was immaterial: what is important is how the body performs sexually (Holland et al., 1998: 116)

indicate that Connell's (1987: 83) understanding of the men as receiving masculinity through social practice may depend on the body of the other for its meaning. For instance, Holland et al. (1996b: 158) found that 'it is only through access to *her* body that a boy can achieve manhood' (my emphasis). Similarly in Gavey et al.'s (1999) research 'some men talked about intercourse as ... something that separates the men from the boys. One male respondent commenting on first heterosex, for instance suggests 'you're not a man till you've had a woman' (1999: 58), while 'other participants indicated that if a [female] partner did not want intercourse it would lead to them feeling "self-doubt"' (1999: 58).

What these findings therefore underline is the significance of embodiment as intercorporeal, indeed that the 'experience of being embodied is never a private affair, but is always already mediated by our continual interactions with other human and non-human bodies' (Weiss, 1999: 5). This is further illustrated by Gough and Edwards's (1998) empirical study of twenty-one-year-old heterosexual men from Manchester. They found:

> that an exclusive focus on the penis per se is unsatisfactory, even when regarded in grandiose terms, ... for it must also be connected to its 'other' – the vagina, and hence penetrative sex ... the penis may only prove significant as a sign of masculinity if connected to its 'legitimate' deployment – heterosexual intercourse ... In this way then, the construction of the penis (as/like masculinity itself) in these extracts is *relational*, and it is that relation that strengthens the heterosexual aspect of hegemonic masculinity. (1998: 417)

In this and the previous study the intercorporeal constitution of sexed differences involves, first, the practice of heterosex, second, the performance of the male body, and, third, to call on Grosz's terms, a 'relational' 'inscription of sexual difference' which takes place through the body of the 'Other':

> The female (or male) body can no longer be regarded as a fixed, concrete substance, a pre-cultural given. It has a determinate form only by being socially inscribed. Each sex is not differentiated on the basis of some unique substance or the possession of distinguishing organs alone. Rather, sexual differences are purely *relational*, each sex being defined only by its negative or differential relations to other sex(es). Out of a spectrum of sexually differential bodies, the continuum is polarised around two sexes, one conceived in terms of the absence, lack or deprivation of the other. (Grosz, 1987: 2)

Grosz's understanding of corporeality as relational and as not concerning the possession of certain organs is taken one step further by Weiss (1999), who points out that the inscription of sexual differences also involves *non-human interaction*, including interactions with medical and mechanical technologies.

Despite Weiss's observation, in the area of AIDS research the focus has been almost exclusively on human interactions. Curiously, social scientists examining safer sex practices have not considered non-human elements of intercorporeality. This is surprising since by definition safer (hetero)sex crucially involves interaction with a non-human object: the condom. And yet the dominant interpretation of condoms in AIDS research assumes that processes of sexual differentiation take place independently of and in opposition to the condom. In this sense AIDS researchers examining safer heterosex practices have taken for granted the condom in their analyses of the body, masculinity and sexual difference. It is to this neglected issue of the condom in AIDS research that I want to turn. In what follows, I show that the condom may be understood following Weiss's thesis on the non-human elements of intercorporeality as central to the constitution of sexual difference.

In a qualitative study of one hundred heterosexual men from New York City, Wyatt-Seal and Ehrhardt (1999) found that the cultural imaginary of condoms and condom use concerned heterosexual men's body maps and identity. Examining heterosexual men and the female condom, Wyatt-Seal and Ehrhardt's (1999) discovered that roughly a quarter of the heterosexually active men they interviewed 'reported complete unwillingness to have sex with a female condom', with some men commenting that 'condom use should be a male domain'. One respondent exclaimed 'nope, I'll stick with mines [the male condom], I don't want to use that'. Whilst a further respondent remarked 'I's the one who uses the condom you understand'. And, according to another, 'I think the man should be using the condom and not the woman' (Wyatt-Seal and Ehrhardt, 1999: 102). Here then the object of the condom reveals not so much women's bodies as the other but rather men's bodies to themselves.

These accounts highlight some of the problems in promoting female condom use in the UK, the US and Australia. Despite an expensive advertising campaign in Britain in 1992, which saw the sales of the Femidon (the British brand name) rise to seventy thousand in ten weeks, the popularity of the female condom had fallen dramatically in 2005 (Burt, 2005: 29). Whilst reasons for the Femidon's unpopularity are understood to result from women's dislike of its shape and noise during sex, Wyatt-Seal and Ehrhardt's findings suggest that heterosexual men may have much to lose in abandoning their control of the (male) condom. Indeed, their findings suggest the condom has been incorporated into our body images and in particular male corporeality and masculine heterosexual subjectivity. These findings thus call into question interpretations of the male condom in safer sex discourse as concerning an 'absent' (Waldby *et al.,* 1991: 39; Richardson, 1990: 173), 'non-existent' (Wilton, 1996: 94) 'invisible' (Richardson, 1996: 173; Wilton, 1996: 95), 'disappearing' (Richardson, 1996: 167) and 'unmarked' heterosexual male body, that is 'not addressed' (Waldby, 1996: 10), and remains 'off-stage'

The condom, gender and sexual difference 115

(Waldby *et al.*, 1993a: 247) and the figuring of women's bodies as unclean, diseased and unsafe (Grosz, 1994; Waldby, 1996). In Weiss's assessment of medical technologies she stresses the 'extent to which they produce and preserve the space of differentiation that makes our intercorporeal exchanges possible' (1999: 128).

Condoms and the making of sexual difference

There is indeed a need to think more carefully about the male condom and the extent to which it produces and preserves the space of differentiation that makes our intercorporeal exchanges possible. In some analyses of empirical research data this has been the case. For instance, in a study of the meaning of condom use for heterosexual men in the 1990s, Waldby, Kippax and Crawford (1993b) consider the way in which the practice of safer heterosex (for heterosexual men) involves the making of a symbolic boundary between different social categories of heterosexual women. Waldby *et al.* (1993b: 35) go on to point out that the practice of differentiating women (via men's 'use of condoms') concerns the constitution of a 'safe' heterosexual masculine self-identity:

> If clean and unclean women can be identified, each young man can create a personal map of infectious and safe relations. Such knowledge permits a hierarchy of infection, in the form of a series of concentric circles, to be inscribed in his social space. He occupies the center and is surrounded by, or surrounds himself with, women whose imagined infectiousness increases as they are allocated positions further and further away. He thus creates an imaginary margin of safety, *a cordon sanitaire*. It is important to note that the perspective of the cordon sanitaire never includes the viewer who occupies its center as an infectious agent, only as a recipient of infection. Furthermore, it is *because the division clean/unclean women is elaborated from the point of view of heterosexual masculinity that it does not include men in its purview as such* ... The dividing of women into two classes is according to their alleged sexual relationships with 'other' men, their bodies as sites shared among a greater or lesser number of men. This division is then used to guide the protocols of condom use. (Waldby *et al.*, 1993b: 31, my emphasis).

But such an interpretation of condom use as concerning a differentiation of *women's bodies* may ignore the significance of condoms for the making of a sexed male body.

In the following account, for instance, the description of a woman as 'unclean' by the male respondent involves the condom:

> Among 'unclean' women, their putative ill-health might be manifest at the site of sex itself, the woman's genitals. Investigating a woman's genitals was a form of precaution. A direct link between promiscuity and diseased genitals is evident in the following anecdote. The woman referred to did not *have* a disease, she is a disease, a body purely for the sexual use of men ... 'I got pretty close [to having sex with her], and – at the last moment, I was no, no way [laughing] no chance. *Didn't have a condom*' ... 'It was a diseased organism' ... 'diseased in the sense that she really was pretty diseasy, if you like, she was sort of pretty raw. An easy diseasy ... I glanced at her, in her vagina, and she was really red and raw and – looking diseased. And I thought, ugh' (Waldby *et al.*, 1993b: 32–33, my emphasis).

Being 'safe' depends not on whether from this respondent's 'point of view' the woman is perceived to be clean or unclean (see Waldby *et al.*, 1993b: 30) but on whether or not *he had a condom* available. Thus whilst the protocols of condom use are understood to involve an inscription of the female body, another way to interpret the condom in this instance is to see it as an extension of a male self.

If the division made in the previous story concerns not so much a distinction between clean and unclean feminine others but, rather, a division between the object of the condom and the other, then the focus on male and female bodies in analyses of safer sex ignores the ways in which the condom concerns the making of sexual difference through processes of self-extension. In Lury's (1998) thesis on *Prosthetic Culture* she argues that self-identity is now constituted as a possession of the individual, a self-possession which she argues is currently being negotiated in a process of experimentation, an experimentation she terms 'prosthetic culture'. What is important for my argument here is that in prosthetic culture the creation of the self does not concern the recognition of Others. Rather, in prosthetic culture, self-identity is constituted through *self-extension*. The adoption or adaption of the condom may therefore be understood as involving the making of sexual difference not through imagining others but as an extension of the self which constitutes a self-possessing individual: that is self-identity. Moreover, if both the object and representation of the condom are understood in this way – as a prosthetic of the self – then we can also question the assumption that sexual difference and a masculine self-identity are produced through natural, fixed or socially determined factors.

If we apply the ideas of the constitution of self-identity through matters of technique, and in particular to my suggestion that in the adoption or adaption of the condom a masculine self-identity is thereby constituted, then we may understand the figuring of male heterosexuality in the context of AIDS to concern the condom. In making this point, I am not suggesting that masculinity precedes the condom, an object which then becomes an extension of the true male self. In other words, I am not assuming, as Munro (1996: 263) warns against in his analysis of extension and identity, that the appropriation of artefacts 'either enlarge or diminish identity'. I am also arguing against dominant understandings of safer sex whereby condom use is assumed to concern the inscription of 'others', and to constitute a threat to a corporeal masculine self-identity, analyses which assume that heterosexual masculinity pre-exists objects like the condom. If, as the previous example illustrates, a distinction between sexed 'male' and sexed 'female' body occurs not through a reflection on the Other but a relation between the self and the object then Haraway's (1991: 201) analysis of 'objects as boundary projects' and of 'embodiment as significant prostheses' (1991: 195) may be helpful for understanding of the history of the condom in AIDS culture.

Where does this account of the condom leave us? In his account of childhood Lee argues that to find that 'all humans are fundamentally dependant on extensions, is not the end of analysis, but the beginning' (2001: 117). In addition Lee stresses that becomings via extension are multiple and sometimes 'come into conflict with one another' (2001: 117). The next chapter analyses some of the consequences of extension. It does so by focusing on the issue of consent in young men's and young women's accounts of the condom in the sexual encounter. By drawing attention to the negotiation of condom use the final chapter shows how consent is disentangled from the person and concerns processes of extension. In so doing I address how such extensions are by no means compatible.

7

Condoms and consent

In November 2003 Marcus Dwayne Dixon, a high school football star, was convicted in Georgia, US, of aggravated child molestation and statutory rape. Dixon was initially charged with raping a classmate, Kristie Brown, in a portable trailer on school property. Brown, who was fifteen at the time of the incident, claimed that she had not consented to intercourse. The fifteen-year-old claimed that the defendant 'tracked her down in a classroom trailer that she was cleaning as part of her duties in an after-school job, asked if she was a virgin, grabbed her arms, unbuttoned her pants and raped her on a table' (cited in Colb, 2004: 2). Dixon, who was eighteen at the time of the incident, claimed that sex was consensual and planned ahead of time. 'The arrangement was for us to go to the trailer, so I put my bag in the car and we went to the trailer and that's where we had sex' (cited in Watson, 2003: 2). The jury agreed with Dixon and acquitted him of rape, sexual battery, aggravated assault and false imprisonment. Because Brown was a virgin, not yet sixteen years old, and Dixon was eighteen, he was convicted of misdemeanour statutory rape and aggravated child molestation, a law that is normally used to protect children from adults and not to police relationships between adolescents. The case attracted much national media attention, not least because of the severity of his ten-year prison sentence, a sentence which in January 2004 was reversed on appeal in the Georgia Supreme Court. Dixon was freed after serving three months in a Georgia prison for having sex with an underage girl.

Most of the controversy surrounding the case, the conviction and the successful appeal concerns race and racial prejudice in the criminal justice system, particularly against black teenagers.

Dixon is an African-American, born to a teenage mother. At the age of nine Dixon was adopted by his white little league coach and wife. Brown, a white southern girl, said 'her daddy was a racist and that he would kill both of us if he knew she was with a black man' (Younge, 2004: 17). Marian Wright Edelman, president of the Children's Defence Fund, argued: 'Marcus's case brings back memories of all the black men who were lynched, executed or imprisoned for having relationships with white women. And it recalls the way black males are perceived to this day' (cited in Younge, 2004: 17). In response, District Attorney Leigh Paterson denied the accusation. 'We believe her story. We believe she was raped. This is not about race. This is about a sexual predator' (cited in Younge, 2004: 17).

The case of Dixon *v.* The State raises many questions regarding adolescence and consent. The issue I want to draw attention to in this case is the significance of the condom. Dixon said he used a condom and threw it away. The investigators said 'they did not look for the condom because they were certain he was not telling the truth. "I didn't believe him an investigator said"' (Younge, 2004: 17). Why? The comment 'I didn't believe him' suggests Dixon was lying. Why were the investigators *certain* Dixon was not telling the truth? Why was Dixon perceived as not capable of using a condom? Why was sex with a condom simply *not possible* for this African American male teenager? If the condom was imagined as an extension of Dixon, would he have been charged with rape? Would the investigators have believed Dixon if he had been a white middle-class adolescent? Could the condom, as an object of evidence, have changed the verdict in the trial? Dixon claimed that sex was planned ahead of time. Having a condom available certainly indicates this is the case. Dixon claimed that the sexual encounter was initiated by the girl. The used condom could indeed suggest that Brown initiated condom use and thus consented to sex. In this instance the condom could have been an extension of herself. But in her account of the rape Brown never mentions the condom. Why? Did she not know? Could the condom have changed her story or the verdict? Why do we not hear her voice in relation to the material evidence of the case? Why does she not make claims on the condom in terms of non-consensual sex? This chapter aims to explore these questions in greater detail. It does so by paying close attention to the similarities and differences in young men's and women's accounts of safer sex in empirical research on condom use. To begin I address the question of consent in the discourse of safer sex.

Consent and the discourse of safer sex

What has been the impact of the 'If it's not on, it's not on' campaign, for instance, on adolescence? One way to address the campaign is as a perlocutionary speech act, that is an education campaign which aimed to incite safer sex as well as a certain kind of (hetero)sexuality. Following Butler we could address the 'If it's not on' campaign as producing certain contextual effects as their consequence, effects that are not necessarily the same thing as the speech act itself and which could give rise to 'speaking in ways that have never been legitimated' (1997: 41). This move contrasts with that made by many AIDS researchers and commentators who consider condom use as an effect of the discourse of safer sex. More specifically, consent is understood within the terms of the utterance 'If it's not on', one which has a performative effect in relation to the condom. But in assuming that the meaning of consent is constituted in the moment of saying 'If the condom is not on I do not consent to having sex with you' AIDS researchers simply map consent on to the condom. In so doing they do not critically address the discourse of safer sex nor the performativity of the condom in the safer sexual encounter. Consider for instance the rape case of Dixon v. The State. The speech act 'I used a condom' was not believed by the investigators. The speech act 'I used a condom' was considered to be a lie and not heard. In this instance the discourse of safer sex and the story of the condom use is not one of equivalence. Dixon's account of his condom use is simply not believed. But what does it imply for this story of condom use to be deemed not credible? What does it mean for his voice not to be heard? Why is Dixon's story of condoms and consent denied? And why does Brown's story of non-consent not include the condom?

Irvine's (2002) history of sex education in the US classroom provides some preliminary answers. Drawing from the work of Austin, *How to Do Things with Words* (1975) and Butler's work *Excitable Speech* (1997), Irvine addresses the impact of the Christian right in opposing comprehensive sex education and campaigning for an abstinence-only curriculum. Opponents of sex education mobilised claims about speech as performative and as having a particular intention. In the 1980s sex education speech is given an illocutionary force and becomes conflated with doing it, sex itself. 'Sex education, they charge, *is* sexual abuse' (2002: 133). Irvine's analysis carefully illustrates how the power of anti-sex-education campaigners was also organised by perlocutionary speech claims whereby the performativity of speech about condoms is literally considered to be lethal to kids. Talk of condoms *will*, it is argued, cause AIDS and murder kids. It is precisely the collapsing of the distinction between words and conduct which, according to Butler (1997), makes possible the kind of state intervention that produced an abstinence-only curriculum in the US. One of the consequences of conflating sex education with child abuse and even the murder of American kids is the shrinking of the discursive space for pleasure and an expansion of sexual danger, fear and shame (Irvine 2002). A further consequence of the abstinence-only curriculum is the shrinking of the discursive space for *consent*, a point well illustrated in the Dixon case.

In the Australian context the policy of comprehensive sex education together with popular safer sex campaigns such as the Grim Reaper advertisement appear to have had a different effect in relation to the performativity of consent. Consider, for instance, the following comments from a young male respondent in Flood's study:

> the main reason I actually had them was, not so much for protection or for um, for any practical purpose but, more so that she couldn't say have you got protection, if you don't no way. *Yeah I've got protection let's go, is that's the reason why I had a condom.* You know so it really didn't bother me if the rubber was a bit perished and it didn't really work properly, because at that stage I wasn't thinking of the implications of pregnancies or diseases or whatever. (Flood, 2000: 260, my emphasis)

In his analysis of safer sex Flood appears to take little notice of what is being said about the condom. But these comments stress the need to address more critically the performativity of consent. In addressing this account we could ask: what role do condoms play in the perfomativity of consent? Is consent necessarily constituted and communicated in language? Is consent a performative effect of safer sex discourse? What role in the sexual encounter does the safer sex discourse play? And what role have sex researchers and social commentators played in producing knowledge about consent in the context of AIDS?

AIDS research, unsafe heterosex and coercion

To consider the role social researchers and theorists have played in creating knowledge about consent let's examine some interpretations of condom use in relation to safer sex education campaigns. The effect of popular advertising campaigns promoting the use of the condom as a way of controlling the transmission of HIV/AIDS and STDs has generally been understood as having a negative outcome in reducing the exchange of bodily fluids because of the social construction of gender. Put simply, gender is seen to have a negative impact on the ability of heterosexual women to achieve safer sex. For example, in the US Patton suggests:

> Monogamy and condom use as promoted in the media are fraught with danger. Women exist in a sexual economy where they have unequal power in relationship to potential sex partners; this inhibits their ability to make a risk evaluation and reasonable changes. (Patton, 1986: 72)

In Britain, Richardson perceives the targeting of heterosexual women in HIV/AIDS health campaigns as doomed to failure:

> articles and pamphlets advise on the importance of safer sex and the use of condoms, but hardly ever do they address the difficulties women may encounter in trying to get their male partners to use condoms and to have safer sex. Nor do they usually analyze why such difficulties occur and how women might respond in such situations. (Richardson, 1990: 170)

These 'difficulties' women face in negotiating safer sex with men are understood to be so great that Richardson argues that the consequences of the discourse of safer sex include the 'issue of women being battered for demanding safer sex and the worry of HIV infection as part of the trauma of having being raped' (Richardson, 1994: 54). Wilton and Aggleton (1991) produce a similar definition of the condom when they suggest that 'women who attempt to negotiate safer sex with male partners risk abuse, physical violence or the loss of that partner' (Wilton and Aggleton, 1991: 155). The point that women who attempt to negotiate safety provoke violent male behaviour is also evident in the work of Heise (1995: 122), who suggests that 'a request for condoms may trigger a violent response'.

What emerges from these accounts is the contradiction between the way women are positioned by the discourse of safer sex and the problem they face in getting men to wear condoms. According to Richardson (1990, 1994, 1996), the gendered structure of heterosexuality (active-male/passive-female), understood to be at play in the context of (hetero)sexual practices, is 'threatened' by the social construction of women as 'active' and in control in the discourse on safer heterosex.

> the construction of normative female sexuality as 'passive' and male as 'active' ... [is] threatened by the allocation of responsibility for negotiating sexual practices to women and the demand that they take active control of the (hetero)sexual encounter. (Richardson, 1996: 174)

The practice of safer sex is thus perceived to be an act through which heterosexual women are able to subvert the gendered dynamic of heterosexuality.

In Holland *et al.*'s research on young women, young men, safer sex and heterosexuality they too interpret the use of condoms in their research findings as positive compared with men's attempts to practise unsafe heterosex. This is the case, they argue, since 'condom use is problematic in that it necessitates a direct confrontation with male power' (Holland *et al.*, 1992a: 155). The interpretation of male power as embodied in the act of heterosex *without* the condom is further elaborated in the work of Wilton, who claims that 'the practice of unsafe sex is, I suggest of a piece with queer bashing, rape [and] ... "rigid gender demarcations" in that it is fundamental to the project of masculinity' (Wilton, 1997: 33). Here then, Wilton extends her analysis of the project of hegemonic masculinity to include unsafe sex, a practice she associates with the act of rape. Sexual coercion in Wilton's analysis thus concerns the literal body part of the penis. Indeed male power according to Wilton and Aggleton is:

> displaced onto that visible and given symbol of innate maleness, the

penis, and onto practices which label and disempower those who are *other* ... Sexual penetration by the penis thereby becomes the symbolic assertion of male power over [the] disempowered other. (Wilton and Aggleton, 1991: 154)

Since their account of male power focuses on the penis, Wilton and Aggleton (1991) and Wilton (1997) produce an account of sexual coercion which simultaneously problematises the male body and normalises the condom.

Safer sex as empowerment?

The normalisation of the condom in sex research and empirical analyses of gender and heterosexuality is further evident in Holland *et al.*'s description of the ways in which young women are perceived to potentially resist male power in a (hetero)sexual context. Although Holland *et al.* point out that

> In the context of sexual encounters, empowering women could mean: not engaging in sexual activity; not engaging in sexual activity without informed consent; *getting men to consent to safer practices* (Holland *et al.*, 1992a: 145, my emphasis)

they do not include the act of women consenting to safer heterosex. In other words Holland *et al.* do not consider the condom as something which women may desire, consent to or actively resist. Their primary focus on men's reluctance to engage in safer practices prevents a consideration of the experience of consent and the condom for young women in the (hetero)sexual encounter.

An understanding of empowerment for young women as involving condom use is however questioned by Moore and Rosenthal's (1991) Australian research findings. They found that the 'say no' factor for their young female respondents was not specifically tied up with refusing to engage in unsafe sex; that is heterosex *without* condoms. Instead Moore and Rosenthal (1991) found that the 'say no' factor for their female respondents involved the act of saying 'no' to safer heterosex; that is sex *with* a condom. Put differently, the heterosexual women in their study did not so much resist men's desire to practise unsafe sex, but also men's desire to practise *safer* sex:

> Women may be accepting the line that sex with a condom is like having a shower with a raincoat ... If males are gradually being

convinced about condom use, they may need to do some convincing of their female partners. (Moore and Rosenthal, 1991: 223)

These women's anti-condom sentiments are analysed in terms of a logic of gender reversal in that the popular 'line' of the condom as interfering with male sexual pleasure – 'like having a shower with a raincoat' – becomes disassociated from young men's account of condom use, and is instead used to describe women's anti-condom sentiments. Consequently Moore and Rosenthal (1991) suggest it is now men who need 'to do some convincing of their female partner' rather than women who must insist on safer sex.

In Holland et al.'s (1998) study, young women's negative descriptions of condom use 'as going to bed with your wellingtons on' are interpreted as concerning the prioritisation of male sexual pleasure:

> The young women report a wide range of negative descriptions of condom use which seem to reflect male perceptions: 'like picking your nose with a rubber glove', 'going to bed with your wellingtons on', 'washing your feet with your socks on'. Although these perceptions were not necessarily presented as male, they nevertheless serve to privilege male sexual pleasure. (Holland et al., 1998: 40)

Whilst these young women's anti-condom sentiments were initially understood by Holland et al. (1998: 43) as reflecting a 'public/male discourse of condoms as passion killers', further questioning by the researchers revealed that the comment 'like having a bath with a raincoat' was for a particular female respondent not about the negative physical experience of condom use for her male partner but rather about her own negative experience of safer heterosex:

> She later said that sex had been painful at first but that after the third time it got better which, she explained, meant that it had stopped hurting. This comment was made well into the interview and it seems it had been easier to initially draw on the public/male discourse of condoms as passion killers. She went on to say that she and her boyfriend did not talk about sex and she *felt unable to tell him what she liked sexually* ... 'I just let him carry on with it.' (Holland et al., 1998: 43, my emphasis)

Read together with Moore and Rosenthal's (1991) findings where young women described their anti-condom sentiments as 'like having a shower whilst wearing a raincoat', these comments suggest that the use of the 'public/male discourse of condoms as passion killers' may in some instances constitute a discourse of *resistance* to condom use.

In Gavey *et al.*'s research, the view of condoms as 'passion killers' for several of the female respondents concerns the condoms interference with women's sexual pleasure. Condoms 'tend to limit what is possible sexually, making sex more predictable, less spontaneous, playful and varied' (Gavey *et al.*, 2001: 929). In analysing their research findings Gavey *et al.* conclude: 'condoms seem to reinforce the coital imperative in two interconnected ways, both in terms of their symbolic reinforcement of the discursive construction of sex as *coitus* and through their material characteristics that contribute at a more practical level to rendering sex as finished after coitus', (Gavey *et al.*, 2001: 928). In addressing safer sex 'in relation to some of the complex gender dynamics that saturate heterosexual encounters', Gavey *et al.* (2001: 918) position the condom as socially disempowering for heterosexual women. What I want to draw out here is the way such an interpretation of the condom, which focuses on the *social impact* of safer sex discourses, does not engage with the *sexual encounter* itself. Nor does it engage with 'the significance of what people may be saying and doing with their [sex] talk' (Widdicombe and Wooffitt, 1995: 65, cited in Speer, 2005: 191).

One reason why women's voices are not always heard and not visible in AIDS research, according to K. Griffin, is the tendency to reduce the concept of empowerment to condom use and especially the 'power to negotiate condom–use' (K. Griffin, 1998: 152). Women who express ambivalent views regarding condom use, especially in relation to heterosex and affective intimacy, 'are not being recognized as a legitimate expression of female subjects' sexual desire' (K. Griffin, 1998: 155) since such ambivalence goes against the logic of AIDS prevention programmes. The problem for heterosexual women is not so much their ability to negotiate the use of condoms but rather the nature of their desire. 'Women who hold these (unrecognized) values are persuaded to adopt condoms in their sexual relations, to the extent that they have been defeated as subjects of female desire, and alienated from their own desires, as they currently understand them' (K. Griffin, 1998: 154). AIDS researchers must therefore move beyond questions of empowerment so as to 'observe a need for positive recognition of female subjects expressed views' (K. Griffin, 1998: 155) and avoid reproducing gendered accounts of both masculine and feminine heterosexualities. There is an urgency in this project since social science research 'is now an important part of the inevitable social construction of desire' (K. Griffin, 1998: 156).

The difficulty in hearing female subjects in AIDS research on condom use is well illustrated in Stewart (1991/92) and in Wyn's (1994) interpretation of Stewart's qualitative research findings. In analysing the response to the question 'would you be worried about what he'd think if you did have one (condom) on you?', both Stewart and Wyn suggest that the social construction of femininity adequately accounts for the following comments from a young female respondent:

> I probably would be, because half of the time sex just happens. You can see a lead up and if I pulled out a condom when things are just starting foreplay it's like saying I'm going to have sex with you now.

According to Stewart:

> Initiating condom use for this young woman presents a major challenge to her definition of femininity and works against her taking the affirmative role which health promotion suggests she should, in negotiating safe sex. (Stewart, 1991/92: 7)

Similarly, Wyn suggests:

> This quotation illustrates the concern that if she were to take out a condom and insist on its use, it would appear to her partner that she had premeditated the scenario, or was too forward or knowledgeable ... The assumption is that her partner would find such an assertion of her sexuality unacceptable. (Wyn, 1994: 35)

But what if something other than femininity is at play here? What if the significance of the condom in the comment 'If I pulled out a condom when things are just starting foreplay it's like saying I'm going to have sex with you now' concerns not so much 'an assertion of her sexuality', an act which 'presents a major challenge to her definition of femininity', but a strategy of delaying heterosex or indeed the communication of consent? Consent in this instance concerns a penetrative imperative. A girl producing a condom suggests 'I want to be penetrated and I want it now', thus curtailing other forms of sexual activity.

What I am suggesting here is that we position the object of the condom as *central* to questions related to consent and its communication, rather than simply focus on the social construction of gender in the discourse of safer sex as an obstacle to young women's pleasure and safety, as is often the case in interpretations of condom use in qualitative research. Holland *et al.*'s analysis illustrates my point:

> Having a condom on one's person indicates a lack of sexual innocence, and the unfeminine identity of a woman actively seeking sex. (Holland *et al.*, 1992b: 278).
>
> Interrupting his performance and being assertive about safety can run counter to being feminine. (Holland *et al.*, 1998: 37)
>
> Feminine identity and expectations of sexual passivity pull against the need to be assertive in order to enjoy sex and ensure personal safety. (Holland *et al.*, 1990b: 343)
>
> reluctance to use condoms came from the women's fear of upsetting men by asserting their own needs. These reasons were partly to do with the fear of losing a boyfriend and the hope of a more committed or steady relationship. (Holland *et al.*, 1991: 139)

By implying that their respondents' reluctance to use condoms primarily concerns the social construction of femininity, which makes these women unwilling to 'be assertive' for 'fear of losing a boyfriend', the researchers are not considering the possibility that these women's ambivalence may concern a resistance to the discourse of safer sex or indeed the communication of non-consent in the sexual encounter. So whilst

> In some cases women had effectively consented to sex, or to unsafe sex, which they did not want, because of what they felt to be *social* pressures, or the importance to them of their relationship or potential relationship with a man (Holland *et al.*,1992c: 654, my emphasis)

the dominant focus on unsafe sex forecloses an analysis of the risky practice of *saying no* to condoms.

The problem of saying no to safer sex is well illustrated in Chan and Fishbein's (1993) study. In their investigation of the determinants of 312 college women's intentions to tell their partners to use condoms, Chan and Fishbein found that, although these women had 'somewhat favourable attitudes toward telling their partners to use condoms' and that 'they intend to tell their partners to use condoms during sexual intercourse', these women perceived themselves to be under 'considerable *normative* pressure to do so' (1993: 1463, my emphasis). The discourse of safer sex could thus be understood as heteronormative, in the sense that it concerns the disciplinary production of gender and heterosexuality and the impossibility of choice whereby the 'subject pursues subordination as the promise of [social] existence' (Butler, 1997: 20).

Saying 'no' to condoms

What I'm looking to highlight here is that whilst the practice of safer heterosex is generally understood as achieving the aims of national and international HIV/AIDS sexual health prevention campaigns, the increased availability of condoms and the normalisation of the act of carrying condoms needs to be addressed more critically. Abbott (1988–89) for example, reports on research findings from an Australian survey conducted in 1986 by the Family Planning Association of Victoria where more than half of the young women surveyed described how they 'would not tell their partner if they were carrying condoms for fear that he may take advantage of them' (1988: 39). Similarly, in Wight's research on young Glaswegian men, he found 'a lack of condoms strengthens women's resistance to initial sexual intercourse' (1993a: 49).

The tension here between the public health discourse of safer (hetero)sex and the issue of consent and its communication is further illustrated in Chapman and Hodgson's (1988) research findings. Two female respondents commenting on the 'image of guys who carry condoms around in their wallets' replied:

> well to me, I'd be put off because its *presumptuous*, but then when I'd stopped and thought about it, at least he's being *careful* in every situation.

> I had a relevantly [*sic*] recent experience where the guy said to me 'hey, I am going to use this' and first of all I thought, *yuk*, but then I thought first *responsible* man that I have met. (Chapman and Hodgson, 1988: 102, my emphases)

These women's perceptions of men initiating condom use as 'presumptuous' and 'yuk' compared with the 'thought' of safer sex as a 'careful' and 'responsible' activity are interpreted by

Chapman and Hodgson as suggesting that 'there is considerable potential to give the condom a symbolism of caring and responsibility' (1988: 104).

Condoms and safer sex?

In an investigation of the relationship between the notion of care and the practice of safer heterosex amongst Australian secondary students (aged sixteen to seventeen), Abbott-Chapman and Denholm (1997) found that for the highest group of condom users (those engaging in first heterosex), the majority of respondents reported that 'caring was not [an] important' (1997: 317) factor in their decision to practise safer heterosex. In other words, the notion of care in this study, as with Kashima et al.'s (1992) findings, was not found to be constituted by the act of young men carrying condoms and using them.

Browne and Minichiello also find in their Australian research that 'male informants found it easier to use condoms when they did *not* care about their partner' (1996: 129). As one male respondent put it, 'I think sometimes sex is just sex, without caring for that person. And that's happened. Then it's not such a big deal that you've got to stop and put it (the condom) on' (1996: 129). In Wight's Scottish study, of the 83 per cent of young men interviewed who said safer sex was using condoms, 'their understanding of the relative HIV risks of different sexual behaviours was largely *irrelevant*' (1994a: 107, my emphasis). In other words, the decision to use condoms was not attributed to the act of taking 'responsibility' for reducing the risks of transmitting HIV. According to Wight (1993b: 475), 'high level of condom use cannot be assumed to be a response to HIV'. And whilst Hillier et al. (1998: 24) find in their research on Australian rural youth evidence of 'the success of the safe sex equals condom message', for the majority of their sample the practice of safer sex was also *not* attributed to reducing the transmission of STD's and HIV/AIDS. On the contrary 'eighty-five percent of [the] sample believed themselves invulnerable' (Hiller et al., 1998: 24). The desire to practise safer heterosex for these adolescent male respondents therefore questions the assumption that condom use is constituted by prior feelings of responsibility for the prevention of sexually tranmissable diseases and HIV. And yet the act of young men carrying condoms and initiating safer sex is often left unaddressed by social researchers in their interpretation of the sexual encounter. This effect, I want to stress, concerns the normalisation of consent in the discourse of safer sex.

Saying 'yes' to condoms

If we consider the discourse of safer sex and in particular the way in which health messages are often concerned with getting women to make *men* agree to condom use, then it seems somewhat implausible that heterosexual women would say no to men's initiation of safer heterosex in AIDS culture. In this sense Gavey's account of how 'women are produced as subjects who are encouraged to regulate our own behavior' (1993: 97) has much to offer for an analysis of safer sex. Gavey's argument that 'women sometimes engage in unwanted sex with men because it does not occur to [them] to question it, but also, sometimes we do not have the *language* to be able to say no' (1993: 102, my emphasis) appears to make some sense of Hillier *et al.*'s findings where at the last intercourse 69 per cent of students (boys 76 per cent, girls 64 per cent) reported that a condom was used, but some of this condom use (37 per cent) 'occurred without negotiation' (1998: 20). The finding that 72 per cent of boys had 'a condom with them at the last sexual encounter' (1998: 21) is interpreted by Hillier *et al.* as 'an established practice in a relationship for a boy using as a matter of course' (1998: 20). Moreover, in Holland *et al.*'s research boys do not consider their desire to practise safer sex to be a problem for young women. A young male respondent comments, 'I mean for all the female people I know, if the bloke says "shall I use a condom?" they say "yes, right, definitely"' (Holland *et al.*, 1998: 44). The 'yes, right, definitely' response indicates that, in both this young man's experience of safer heterosex and through his communication with others, young women do not usually *say no* to the condom. Nor do these men 'generally expect young women to resist their propositions of condom use' (Holland *et al.*, 1998: 34).

The following comments from two women in Browne and Minichiello's (1994) Australian study further highlight the ambiguity of consent in relation to safer sex. 'You talk about it ... but you don't *really* talk about it' (1994: 240). And:

Although it's not carte blanche, it's almost like – well (by deciding to use condoms) – we've agreed to have sex, so if the condom is available and that's worked out with minimal discussion, then that's it by default almost. (Brown and Minichiello, 1994: 241)

The comments that 'you don't *really* talk about it' and condom use just happens 'by default almost' 'with minimal discussion' suggest that the practice of safer sex ultimately concerns the *availability* of the condom.

Indeed, in this study 'having no condom available was problematic to the sexual experience' whilst 'available condoms were seen as a symbolic agreement to penetrative sex which effectively stopped dialogue – by default' (Browne and Minichiello, 1994: 238–239). Browne and Minichiello also note that the practice of safer heterosex 'by default' was constituted through a lack of negotiation. Moreover, they argue that it is heterosexual men who are forced to engage in safer heterosex:

> Men it seems agree to condom use, but this is through agreed, passive compliance rather than active participation and adoption of a 'personal decision to use'. (Brown and Minichiello, 1994: 245–246)

In this account heterosexual men are perceived to occupy a vulnerable position in relation to the *negotiation* of condom use. But such an interpretation is challenged by findings from Wight's study where over a quarter of the male respondents reported that initial acts of safer sex took place in situations where there was 'no negotiation about precautionary behavior' (1993a: 46). One male respondent commented:

> I was not really scared that she would fall pregnant, I was not scared that she would have the virus. I think at the back of my mind [was] that once I pulled my condom out then that meant that I was having sex ... As opposed to lying between her and fumbling and making a mess of it and then her changing her mind. *I felt that if I made that move by putting the condom on then we were at the point of no return.* (Wight, 1993a: 47, my emphasis)

According to Wight, this 'male respondent used condoms as a non-verbal way of clarifying their wish to have sexual intercourse' (1999: 753). Whilst the comment 'once I pulled my condom out then that meant that I was having sex' suggests that the act of producing a condom is constitutive of consent for the male subject, making that move could also reduce the possibility of consent by the female subject.

These comments thus highlight the need to question the gendered experience of condoms and consent in the sexual encounter. In a study on sexual scenarios and the communication of consent by adolescents, Rosenthal (1997) found that for both boys and girls (aged fifteen to seventeen years) 'communication was judged as clearer when the message was yes to sex rather than no' (1997: 489) with 'few differences between boys and girls in reports of the clarity of the messages conveyed' (1997: 490). A surprising finding was the 'divergence of young people's views about what constitutes clear communication, pressure and acceptability' (1997: 489) with communication only 'part of the whole' (1997: 490). Although Moore and Rosenthal (1993) speculate that condom use usually requires that both partners communicate and agree before the behaviour occurs, they also stress that using a condom is not a private act carried out well in advance of a sexual encounter – unlike taking a contraceptive pill. 'The negotiated, shared aspect of using condoms is likely to add considerably to the difficulties in dealing with condoms ... Because of this, the immediate context of the sexual encounter may have a more powerful influence on adolescents' sexual decisions to use a condom than any distal normative influences' (1993: 138).

The point that the decision to use condoms concerns the immediate context of the sexual encounter is well illustrated in the following accounts:

> She didn't even ask ... Just got one from the drawer ... I think it's good because, if you don't mind ... you don't like to be the one to bring it up because you're worried you'll spoil it and you'll miss out ... so it's good if it's easy like that. (Browne and Minichiello, 1994: 238)

> She said, 'you'd better be using a condom'. And that was like, I was ... I was thinking that nothing would happen, and suddenly, 'Do you have a condom?' ... Oh right! Here we go! So I knew from then [that we would have sex]. (Mitchell and Wellings, 2002: 399)

In these accounts the condom is an actor in constitution of consent. Moreover, consent is made possible by the object of the condom. Indeed these accounts highlight the importance of the condom in producing the possibilities of consent. But this in itself presents problems. As a male respondent puts it:

> It's a problem also having condoms. Like if you're meeting out on a first date or something, you don't want to take condoms along, cos if she did see them she would be saying, 'What are you doing?' and you'd be going, 'Just in case', you know, I'm not saying ... (Mitchell and Wellings, 2002: 402)

Such a strategy was found to be inappropriate in the sexual encounter as it was perceived to reduce young women's options and the ability to say no to sex 'since talking about condoms is perceived as tantamount to assuming sex will occur' (Mitchell and Wellings, 2002: 405). Empirical interpretations of condom use which position the condom as either empowering or disempowering for young heterosexual women (and men) are thus unable to address the performativity of consent in relation to the condom since they measure condom use externally, that is, outside of the sexual encounter.

A young woman from Warr's (2001) research, for instance, comments: 'He just gave me [a condom] and went "here", and I thought oh, cool, he's a safety boy, this is all right' (2001: 250). In this instance communication is limited and the condom is desired in the context of the sexual encounter. But in her analysis of this young woman's comments Warr foregrounds the social meaning of condoms and in particular 'a notion of "romantic safe sex" because romance with its references to the emotional qualities of love, intimacy and reciprocity remains highly pleasurable' for women (2001: 242). In so doing Warr maps the social construction of gender and heterosexuality onto the condom, a move which reproduces the social rather than challenging it. The following comments from a female respondent further illustrate the problem with such interpretations of safer sex:

> one night we went back to his house, and he didn't really force me, but I didn't really want to, *but I did want to*. And I was really frightened. And I remember saying – we can't do it because I might get pregnant. And he got these condoms out, and that was it then. I was sort of frightened but not frightened. (Holland *et al.*, 1990a: 134, my emphasis)

Whilst the remark 'he got the condoms out, and that was it then' could be interpreted as indicating that this particular woman's feelings of ambivalence were somewhat resolved 'when he got these condoms out', the comment 'that was it then' suggests the meaning of consent is here detached from the person and concerns the condom. This account thus illustrates how social interpretations of safer sex are in fact re-essentialising of gender. That is, they position gender as 'a fixed trait residing in the individual speaker rather than a social construct located in interaction' (Speer, 2005: 60). Consequently they are unable to address the way gender is not so much imposed from outside of the sexual context but is rather constituted within it. By focusing on the practice of safer sex this chapter has shown that consent could be better understood in relation to the condom itself, an object which constitutes the adolescent subject in ways that may not always be heard, but need to be legitimised. If the condom creates the possibility of consent, social researchers, sex educators and criminal investigators must be open to this possibility.

Conclusion: condoms, adolescence and time

I began with a speculative question of how to address the history of the condom. How to make sense of safer sex discourse? In addressing this question I have argued that what is at stake is not whether it makes sense to refer to the condom in the context of AIDS as making visible or indeed invisible certain sexualities. Rather *Object Matters* has shown how the condom concerns the production and regulation of heterosexuality.

My analysis of empirical data in Chapters 5 and 6 showed how the intelligibility of sexed bodies, gender identity and heterosexuality is not compromised or even contested by safer sex discourse. Instead I pointed out how the practice of safer sex is a moment in time that marks experience. In particular, the first time is crucial for the way in which young men and women see themselves and each other. In this instance the condom is constitutive of a corporeal male body-image and masculine gender identity.

But at the same time *Object Matters* has cautioned the reader against naturalising the performativity of the condom. This is the case, it was argued, because the condom produces a naturalisation of time in relation to sexuality. In Chapters 2 and 3 it was shown how the logic of safer sex concerns a narrative of development, responsibility and a transition to adult (hetero)sexuality. I pointed out that the temporality of the condom as future-oriented involves the governing of populations and sexual identities, and in particular adolescent sexuality. Adolescence should therefore be understood not as a transitional time or indeed an in-between time but as a sexual category that involves specific modes of regulation. What this book draws attention to is the significance of the condom for the regulation of future-oriented adolescent (hetero)sexuality.

Conclusion 137

This book has also questioned the narration of AIDS during a particular time of the epidemic. Examining the period 1986–96 I considered how a range of actors including social government, social scientists, social theorists and young people themselves responded to the AIDS crisis. Throughout the chapters I showed the extent to which these actors have all been participants in the historiography of the condom. In this sense I have offered an alternative history of AIDS.

In Chapters 5 and 6 I questioned the view that the advent of AIDS and the discourse of safer sex constituted a crisis in masculinity for heterosexual men. Here it was shown that feminists responding to the mainstreaming of safer sex discourse perceived the change brought by AIDS in the mid-1980s as one which threatened and challenged phallocentricism, deprivileged heterosexism and denaturalised male embodiment. I demonstrated that these views worked towards creating knowledge on condom use as deconstructing the social, particularly normative gender and sexual identities. At the same time it was shown how this deconstructive logic failed to recognise the ways in which the performativity of the condom concerns processes of male self-extension and the constitution of a masculine heterosexual self-identity (Chapter 6). So, although these theoretical analyses have transformative effects in relation to the meaning of the condom, my goal in Chapter 5 was to describe how such historical accounts of safer sex as transforming, subverting and challenging phallocentricism and heterosexism naturalise – rather than historicise – the category of heterosexuality and male gender identity.

In Chapter 3 I examined the consequences of AIDS research on condom use. In particular, I examined the assumption that qualitative research methods are more adept at capturing people's sexual experiences. I also questioned the assumption that non-statistical methods can produce knowledge of non-normative sexual practices and sexualities. In the context of AIDS I argued that social research on adolescent condom use nonetheless produces normative accounts of heterosexuality. This occurs for a number of reasons. Throughout the 1990s funding for AIDS social research was geared towards adolescents even though this group was a low-risk group in relation to HIV. The problem with getting adolescents to talk about safer sex is that it takes this category for granted. And yet, as Gordon points out, adolescence is a temporal category which is geared towards a (hetero)sexual future. In attempting to measure the relationship between the social change brought about by AIDS and adolescent condom use, social researchers thus naturalise heterosexuality as an imminent futurity. A further consequences of getting young people to speak about condoms is that such stories render the adolescent a sexual subject with a particular future-oriented (hetero)sexual self-identity.

While the condom concerns the production of a future (sexual) self, this book has explored the ways it can also stop time. For example, in Chapters 2 and 4, I illustrated the ways in which assumptions about race, class and ethnicity impact on the way social researchers, social theorists and sex educators interpret safer sex. White middle-class adolescents are considered to respond to safer sex messages and change their future behaviour accordingly whereas working-class, black and ethnic kids are not considered to have the capacities to do so. The assumption here is that some kids lack a future-oriented sexual subjectivity. In this way the condom disrupts the narrative of adolescence as a movement from the present to future (hetero)sexual adulthood. These assumptions about safer sex are also reflected in the views of young people themselves. In Chapter 4 I showed how safer sex is interpreted as a white person's kind of awareness and a practice associated with white middle-class adolescents. In describing how the condom becomes an extension of white adolescence and a marker of difference I demonstrated that adolescence is not an ontological given or natural category but a sexual category which produces social divisions along the lines of race, class and ethnicity.

In analysing AIDS research on safer sex this book has drawn attention to a further set of issues regarding the condom. In Chapter 7 it was pointed out that the practice of safer heterosex is normalised in qualitative research. This is the case because social researchers and social theorists have assumed that unsafe sex is problematic in the context of AIDS whilst safer sex is assumed to involve practices of self-responsibility, care and the negotiation of safety. In so doing AIDS researchers have focused on the practice of *unsafe* sex in their analyses of empirical research findings. As a result the condom is left unaddressed. By drawing attention to the place of the condom in adolescent safer sex stories I suggested that social researchers have overlooked the fundamental issue of consent. Instead of assuming that condom use is consensual, as is normally the case, I argued the condom itself constitutes the possibility of choice and consent. But at the same time it was shown that the logic of safer sex reduces the possibility of consent.

How then should we understand the history of the condom? We should, I suppose, look to the past. By looking to the past this book has shown how the future has been a constant theme in attempts to educate the public about sex (see Chapters 2 and 4). My reading of texts outlining sex education discourse in school education policies and public health campaigns in three different national cultures has drawn attention to this particular historical pattern. I have shown that the emphasis on sexual self-control, morality and individual responsibility in sex education discourse concerns the regulation of an adolescent's (hetero)sexual future. In the context of AIDS I have suggested that the discourse of safer sex produces a new modality of regulation which concerns the category of adolescence *and* the object of the condom. In this sense *Object Matters* has produced an interpretative history of the condom as one which connects the present with the past. Whilst the history of the condom outlined in this book could be read as concerning the transformation of the objects meaning in time, it can also be read in relation to the temporality of the object. Focusing on the period 1986–96 I have argued that the temporality of the condom concerns the making of future generations, the future of the nation and the future itself. This transformation has considerable consequence for how we live our lives and the choices we make. The more clearly we come to understand the temporality of the condom as a prolongation of the present into the future, the more it will become possible to make the future different.

References

Abbott, S. (1988–89), 'AIDS and young women', *The Bulletin of the National Clearinghouse for Youth Studies*, 7:4–8, 38–41.

Abbott-Chapman, J. and C. Denholm (1997), 'Adolescent risk taking and the romantic ethic: HIV/AIDS awareness in Yr. 11 & 12 students', *The Australian and New Zealand Journal of Sociology*, 33:3, 306–322.

Adkins, L. (2002), *Revisions: Sexuality and Gender in Late Modernity* (Buckingham: Open University Press).

Altman, D. (1995), 'Meanings and identities in the time of AIDS', in R. G. Parker and J. H. Gagnon (eds), *Conceiving Sexuality: Approaches to Sex Research in a Postmodern World* (New York and London: Routledge), pp. 97–108.

Ang, I. (1995), '"I'm a feminist but..." "Other" women and postnational feminism', in B. Caine and R. Pringle (eds), *Transitions: New Australian Feminisms* (New York: St Martin's Press), pp. 57–73.

Austin, J. L. (1975), *How to Do Things and Words* (Cambridge, MA, and London: Harvard University Press).

Bashford, A. (2004), *Imperial Hygiene: A Critical History of Colonialism, Nationalism, and Public Health* (Basingstoke and New York: Macmillan Press).

Berlant, L. (1997), *The Queen of America Goes to Washington City* (Durham and London: Duke University Press).

Berridge, V. (1996), *AIDS in the UK: The Making of Policy 1981–1994* (Oxford: Oxford University Press).

Bersani, L. (1988), 'Is the rectum a grave?', in D. Crimp (ed.), *AIDS: Cultural Analysis, Cultural Activism* (Cambridge, MA: MIT Press), pp. 197–224.

Bland, L. (1982), '"Guardians of the race", or "Vampires upon the nation's health"?: female sexuality and its regulation in early twentieth-century Britain', in E. Whitelegg (ed.), *The Changing Experience of Women* (Buckingham: Open University Press), pp. 373–388.

Bland, L. (1996), 'The shock of the freewoman journal: feminists speaking on heterosexuality in early twentieth-century England', in J. Weeks and J. Holland (eds), *Sexual Cultures: Communities, Values and Intimacy* (London: Macmillan), pp. 75–97.

Bordo, S. (1994), 'Reading the male body', in L. Goldstein (ed.), *The Male Body* (Michigan: University of Michigan Press), pp. 265–306.

Bordo, S. (1997), *Twighlight Zone* (Berkeley: University of California Press).

Braidotti, R. (1997), 'Remembering Fitzroy High', in J. Mead (ed.), *Bodyjamming: Sexual Harassment, Feminism and Public Health* (Sydney: Vintage), pp. 121–147.

Brandt, A. M. (1987), *No Magic Bullet: A Social History of Venereal Disease in the United States since 1880* (Oxford: Oxford University Press).

Bravmann, S. (1991), '(Almost) nothing queer here: comments on Joshua Gamson's "Rubber Wars"', *Journal of the History of Sexuality*, 2:1, 98–102.

Bray, F. and S. Chapman (1991), 'Community knowledge, attitudes and media recall about AIDS, Sydney 1988 and 1989', *Australian Journal of Public Health*, 15:2, 107–113.

Brown, W. (1995), *States of Injury: Power and Freedom in Late Modernity* (Princeton: Princeton University Press).

Browne, J. and V. Minichiello (1994), 'The condom: why more people don't put one on', *Sociology of Health & Illness*, 16:2, 229–251.

Browne, J. and V. Minichiello (1996), 'Condoms: dilemmas of caring and autonomy in heterosexual safe sex practices', *Venereology*, 9:1, 24–32.

Burt, K. (2005), 'What happened to the Femidom?', *Guardian Weekly*, 2–8 September, p. 29.

Buston, K. and D. Wight (2002), 'The salience and utility of school sex education to young women', *Sex Education*, 2:3, 233–250.

Buston, K. and D. Wight (2006), 'The salience and utility of school sex education to young men', *Sex Education*, 6:2, 135–150.

Buston, K., D. Wight and S. Scott (2001), 'Difficulty and diversity: the context and practice of sex education', *British Journal of the Sociology of Education*, 22, 353–368.

Butler, J. (1990), *Gender Trouble: Feminism and the Subversion of Identity* (New York and London: Routledge).

Butler, J. (1992), 'The lesbian phallus and the morphological imaginary', *Differences: A Journal of Feminist Cultural Studies*, 4:1, 133–171.

Butler, J. (1993), *Bodies that Matter: On the Discursive Limits of 'Sex'* (New York and London: Routledge).

Butler, J. (1997), *Excitable Speech: A Politics of the Performative* (New York and London: Routledge).

Campbell, C. (2003), *Letting Them Die: Why HIV/AIDS Prevention Programmes Fail* (Oxford: James Currey, Bloomington: Indiana University Press).

Campbell, C., Y. Nair and S. Maimane (2006), 'AIDS stigma, sexual moralities and the policing of women and youth in South Africa', *Feminist Review*, 83, 132–138.

Carter, J. B., 'Birds bees, and venereal disease: towards an intellectual history of sex education', *Journal of the History of Sexuality*, 10, 213–249.

Chan, D. K.-S. and M. Fishbein (1993), 'Determinants of college women's intentions to tell their partners to use condoms', *Journal of Applied Social Psychology*, 23:18, 1455–1470.

Chapman, S. and J. Hodgson (1988), 'Showers in raincoats: attitudinal barriers to condom use in high risk heterosexuals', *Community Health Studies*, 12:1, 97–105.

Chapman, S., L. Stoker, M. Ward, D. Porritt and P. Fahey (1990), 'Discriminant attitudes and beliefs about condoms in young multi-partner heterosexuals', *International Journal of STD & AIDS*, 1, 422–428.

Chapman-DeBro, S., S. M. Campbell and L. A. Peplau (1994), 'Influencing a partner to use a condom', *Psychology of Women Quarterly*, 18, 165–182.

Church-Gibson, P. and R. Gibson (1993), *Dirty Looks: Women, Pornography, Power* (London: BFI Publishing).

Cohen, C. (1999), *The Boundaries of Blackness: AIDS and the Breakdown of Black Politics* (Chicago: University of Chicago Press).

Colb, S. (2004), 'The pros and cons of statutory rape laws: a ten year sentence for Marcus Dwayne Dixon', CNN.com, 13 February, 1–4.

Connell, R. W. (1987), *Gender and Power: Society, the Person and Sexual Politics* (Cambridge: Polity Press).

Connell, R. W. (1995), *Masculinities* (St Leonards: Allen and Unwin).

Conway, M. T. (1996), 'Inhabiting the phallus: reading Safe As Desire', *Camera Obscura: Feminist Culture and Media Studies*, 38 (May), 133–160.

Coward, R. (1982), 'Sexual violence and sexuality', *Feminist Review*, 11 (June), 9–22.

Coward, R. (1984), *Female Desire* (London: Granada Publishers).

Coward, R. (1987), 'Sex after AIDS', *New Internationalist*, 20 March, 11–12.

Crawford, J., A. Turtle and S. Kippax (1990), 'Student-favoured strategies for AIDS avoidance', *Australian Journal of Psychology*, 42:2, 123–137.

Crawford, J., S. Kippax and C. Waldby (1994), 'Women's sex talk and

men's sex talk: different worlds', *Feminism and Psychology*, 4:4, 571–587.
Crawford, R. (1994), 'The boundaries of the self and the unhealthy other: reflections on health, culture and AIDS', *Social Science and Medicine*, 38:10, 1347–1365.
Cronin, A. M. (2000a), 'Consumerism and compulsory individuality', in S. Ahmed, J. Kilby, C. Lury, M. McNeill and B. Skeggs (eds), *Transformations: Thinking Through Feminism* (London and New York: Routledge), pp. 273–287.
Cronin, A. M. (2000b), *Advertising and Consumer Citizenship: Gender, Images and Rights* (London and New York: Routledge).
Dean, T. (2000), *Beyond Sexuality* (Chicago and London: The University of Chicago Press).
D'Emilio, J. and E. B. Freedman (1997), *Intimate Matters: A History of Sexuality in America* (Chicago: University of Chicago Press, 2nd edition).
Dowsett, G. W. (1996), *Practicing Desire: Homosexual Sex in the Era of AIDS* (Stanford: Stanford University Press).
Dunne, M., J. Lucke, R. Nilsson and B. Raphael (1993), *National HIV/AIDS Evaluation 1992 HIV Risk and Sexual Behaviour Survey in Australian Secondary Schools* (Canberra: Commonwealth Department of Health and Community Studies).
Durham, M. (1991), *Sex and Politics: The Family and Morality in the Thatcher Years* (Basingstoke and London: Macmillan Press).
Dworkin, A. (1981), *Pornography: Men Possessing Women* (London: The Women's Press).
Dyer, R. (1982), 'Don't look now – the male pin up', *Screen*, 23:3–4, 61–73.
Dyer, R. (1985), 'Male gay porn: coming to terms', *Jump Cut*, 30, 27–29.
Dyer, R. (1993), *The Matter of Images* (London and New York: Routledge).
Edelman, L. (2004), *No Future: Queer Theory and the Death Drive* (Durham and London: Duke University Press).
Ericksen, J. A. (1999), *Kiss and Tell: Surveying Sex in the Twentieth Century* (Cambridge, MA, and London: Harvard University Press).
Fenton S. and K. Charsley (2000), 'Epidemiology and sociology as incommensurate games: accounts from the study of health and ethnicity', *Health*, 4:4, 403–425.
Ferguson, R. (2000), 'The nightmares of the heteronormative', *Cultural Values*, 4:4, 419–444.
Findlay, H. (1992), 'Freud's "fetishism" and the lesbian dildo debates', *Feminist Studies*, 18:3, 563–580.
Flood, M. (2000), *Lust, Trust and Latex: Young Heterosexual Men and*

Condom Use (Unpublished PhD thesis, Department of Women's Studies, Australian National University, Canberra).

Flowers, P. (2001), 'Gay men and HIV/AIDS risk management', *Health*, 5:1, 50–75.

Foucault, M. (1978), *The History of Sexuality: Volume 1* (London: Penguin Books).

Franklin, S., C. Lury and J. Stacey (2000), *Global Nature, Global Culture* (London and New Delhi: Sage).

Fraser, M. (1999), *Identity without Selfhood: Simone de Beauvoir and Bisexuality* (London: Cambridge University Press).

Fung, R. (1991), 'Looking for my penis: the eroticised Asian in gay male porn', in Bad Object Choices (ed.), *How Do I Look?* (Seattle: Bay Press).

Fuqua, J. V. (1995), '"There's a queer in my soap!": the homophobia/AIDS story-line of One Life To Live', in R. Allen (ed.), *To Be Continue . . . Soap Operas Around the World* (London and New York: Routledge), pp. 199–213.

Fuss, D. (1991), 'Inside/out', in D. Fuss (ed.), *Inside/out* (London and New York: Routledge), pp. 1–12.

Gagnon, J. H. and W. Simon (1970), *The Sexual Scene* (Chicago: Aldine).

Gallois, C., D. Terry, P. Timmins, Y. Kashima and M. McCamish (1994), 'Safe sexual intentions and behaviour among heterosexuals and homosexual men: testing the theory of reasoned action', *Psychology and Health*, 1:10 (1994), 1–16.

Gamson, J. (1990), 'Rubber Wars: struggles over the condom in the United States', *Journal of the History of Sexuality*, 1:2, 262–282.

Gamson, J. (1991), 'Gamson's response to Trumbach and Bravmann', *Journal of the History of Sexuality*, 2:1, 102–105.

Gavey, N. (1993), 'Technologies and effects of heterosexual coercion', in S. Wilkinson and C. Kitzinger (eds), *Heterosexuality: A Feminism and Psychology Reader* (London: Sage).

Gavey, N., K. McPhillips and V. Braun (1999), '*Interruptus coitus*: heterosexuals accounting for intercourse', *Sexualities*, 2:1, 35–68.

Gavey, N., K. McPhillips and M. Doherty (2001), '"If it's not on, it's not on" – or is it? Discursive constraints on women's condom use', *Gender & Society*, 15:6, 917–934.

Gilman, S. L. (1988), *Disease and Representation: Images of Illness from Madness to Disease* (Ithaca and London: Cornell University Press).

Gordon, A. (1999), 'Turning back: adolescence, narrative and queer theory', *GLQ*, 5:1, 1–24.

Gott, T. (1997), 'Sex and the single T-cell: the taboo of HIV-positive sexuality in Australian art and culture', in J. J. Matthews (ed.), *Sex in Public* (Sydney: Allen and Unwin), pp. 139–156.

Gough B. and G. Edwards (1998), 'The beer talking: Four lads, a carry out and the reproduction of masculinities', *The Sociological Review*, 46:3, 409–435.

Griffin, G. (1998), 'Safe and sexy: lesbian erotica in the age of AIDS', in L. Pearce and J. Stacey (eds), *Romance Revisited* (London: Lawrence and Wishart), pp. 129–157.

Griffin, K. (1998), 'Beyond empowerment: heterosexualities and the prevention of AIDS', *Social Science and Medicine*, 46:2, 151–156.

Grosz, E. (1987), 'Notes towards a corporeal feminism', *Australian Feminist Studies*, 5 (Summer), 1–16.

Grosz, E. (1990), 'Inscriptions and body-maps: representations and the corporeal', in T. Threadgold and A. Cranny-Francis (eds), *Feminine/Masculine/Representation* (St Leonards: Allen and Unwin), pp. 62–74.

Grosz, E. (1994), *Volatile Bodies* (St Leonards: Allen and Unwin).

Hage, G. (1998), *White Nation: Fantasies of White Supremacy in a Multicultural Society* (Annandale: Pluto Press).

Halberstam, J. (1994), 'F2M: the making of female masculinity', in L. Doan (ed.), *The Lesbian Postmodern* (New York: Columbia University Press), pp. 210–228.

Halberstam, J. (1997), 'Techno-homo: on bathrooms, butches, and sex with furniture', in J. Terry and M. Calvert (eds), *Processed Lives: Gender and Technology in Everyday Life* (New York and London: Routledge), pp. 183–194.

Hall, G. S. (1904), *Adolescence* (New York: Appleton).

Hall, L. A. (1991), *Hidden Anxieties: Male Sexuality 1900–1950* (Oxford: Polity).

Hall, L. A. (2004), 'Eyes tightly shut, lying rigidly still, and thinking of England? British women and sex from Marie Stopes to Hite 2000', in C. Nelson and M. Martin (eds), *Sexual Pedagogies: Sex Education in Britain, Australia and America* (New York and England: Palgrave Macmillan), pp. 53–71.

Hammonds, E. (1986), 'Race, sex and AIDS: the construction of the "Other"', *Radical America*, 20:6, 28–36.

Hampshire, J. A. (2005), 'The politics of school sex education policy in England and Wales from the 1940s to the 1960s', *Social History of Medicine*, 18:1, 87–105.

Haraway, D. (1991), *Simians, Cyborgs and Women* (London and New York: Routledge).

Harre, R. (2002), 'Material objects in social worlds', *Theory, Culture & Society*, 19:5/6, 23–33.

Heise, L. (1995) 'Violence, sexuality and women's lives', in R. G. Parker and J. H. Gagnon (eds), *Conceiving Sexuality: Approaches to Sex*

Research in a Postmodern World (London and New York: Routledge), pp. 109–134.

Hillier, L., L. Harrison and D. Warr (1998), '"When you carry condoms all the boys think you want it": negotiating competing discourses about safe sex', *Journal of Adolescence*, 21, 15–29.

Holland, J., C. Ramazanoglu and S. Scott (1990a), 'Managing risk and experiencing danger: tensions between government AIDS education policy and young women's sexuality', *Gender and Education*, 2:2, 125–145.

Holland, J., C. Ramazanoglu and S. Scott, S. Sharpe and R. Thomson (1990b), 'Sex, gender and power; young women's sexuality in the shadow of AIDS', *Sociology of Health & Illness*, 12:3, 336–350.

Holland, J., C. Ramazanoglu, S. Scott, S. Sharpe and R. Thomson (1990c), *'Don't die of ignorance' – 'I nearly died of embarrassment': Condoms in Context* (London: The Tufnell Press).

Holland, J., C. Ramazanoglu, S. Scott, S. Sharpe and R. Thomson (1991), 'Between embarrassment and trust: young women and the diversity of condom use', in P. Aggleton, G. Hart and P. Davies (eds), *AIDS: Responses, Interventions and Care* (London: The Falmer Press), pp. 127–148.

Holland, J., C. Ramazanoglu, S. Scott, S. Sharpe and R. Thomson (1992a), 'Pressure, resistance, empowerment: young women and the negotiation of safer sex', in P. Aggleton, P. Davies and G. Hart (eds), *AIDS: Rights, Risk and Reason* (London: The Falmer Press), pp. 142–163.

Holland, J., C. Ramazanoglu, S. Sharpe and R. Thomson (1992b), 'Risk, power and the possibility of pleasure: young women and safer sex', *AIDS Care*, 4:3, 273–283.

Holland, J., C. Ramazanoglu, S. Sharpe and R. Thomson (1992c), 'Pleasure, pressure and power: some contradictions of gendered sexuality', *Sociological Review*, 40:4, 645–674.

Holland, J., C. Ramazanoglu, S. Sharpe and R. Thomson (1994), 'Power and desire: the embodiment of female sexuality', *Feminist Review*, 46, 21–38.

Holland, J., C. Ramazanoglu, S. Sharpe and R. Thomson (1996a), 'Reputations: journeying into gendered power relations', in J. Weeks and J. Holland (eds), *Sexual Cultures: Communities, Values and Intimacy* (Basingstoke: Macmillan), pp. 239–260.

Holland, J., C. Ramazanoglu and R. Thomson (1996b), 'In the same boat? The gendered inexperience of first heterosex', in D. Richardson (ed.), *Theorising Heterosexuality: Telling It Straight* (Buckingham: Open University Press), pp. 143–160.

Holland, J., C. Ramazanoglu, S. Sharpe and R. Thomson (1998), *The*

Male in the Head (London: The Tufnell Press).
Hollway, W. (1984), 'Women's power in heterosexual sex', *Women's Studies International Forum*, 7:1, 63–68.
Irvine, J. (2000), 'Doing it with words: discourse and the sex education culture wars', *Critical Inquiry*, 27 (Autumn), 58–76.
Irvine, J. (2002), *Talk about Sex: The Cultural Politics of Sexuality Education* (Berkeley: The University of California Press).
Jackson, S. (1978), 'How to make babies: sexism in sex education', *Women's Studies International Quarterly*, 1, 341–352.
Jackson, S. (1982), *Childhood and Sexuality* (Oxford: Basil Blackwell).
Jackson, S. and S. Scott (1997), 'Gut reactions to matters of the heart: reflections on rationality, irrationality and sexuality', *Sociological Review*, 15:4, 571–574.
Jagose, A. (2002), *Inconsequence: Lesbian Representation and the Logic of Sexual Sequence* (Ithaca and London: Cornell University Press).
Jeffreys, S. (1990), *Anticlimax* (London: The Women's Press).
Jeffreys, S. (1993), *The Lesbian Heresy* (Melbourne: Spinifex).
Johnston, A. M., J. Wadsworth, K. Wellings and J. Field (1994), *Sexual Attitudes and Lifestyles* (Oxford: Blackwell).
Juffer, J. (1998), *At Home with Pornography: Women, Sex and Everyday Life* (New York and London: New York University Press).
Juhasz, A. (1990), 'The contained threat: women in mainstream AIDS documentary', *The Journal of Sex Research*, 27:1, 25–46.
Kaite, B. (1995), *Pornography and Difference* (Bloomington: Indiana University Press).
Kappeler, S. (1986), *The Pornography of Representation* (Cambridge: Polity Press).
Kashima, Y., C. Gallois and M. McCamish (1992), 'Predicting the use of condoms, past behaviour, norms, and the sexual partner', in T. Edgar, M. A. Fitzpatrick and V. Freimuth (eds), *AIDS: A Communication Perspective* (London: Lawrence Erlbaum).
Kimmel, M. S. (1990), 'After fifteen years: the impact of the sociology of masculinity on the masculinity of sociology', in J. Hearn and D. Morgan (eds), *Men, Masculinities and Social Theory* (London: Unwin Hyman), pp. 93–109.
Kimmel, M. S. and M. P. Levine (1992), 'Men and AIDS', in M. S. Kimmel and M. A. Messner (eds), *Men's Lives* (New York: Macmillan, 2nd edn), pp. 318–329.
Kipnis, L. (1996), *Bound and Gagged: Pornography and the Politics of Fantasy in America* (New York: Grove Press).
Kippax, S., J. Crawford, C. Waldby and P. Benton (1990), 'Women negotiating heterosex: implications for AIDS prevention', *Women's Studies International Forum*, 13:6, 533–542.

Kippax, S. and P. Kinder (2002), 'Reflexive practice: the relationship between social research and health promotion HIV prevention', *Sex Education*, 2:2, 91–104.

Kroker, A. and M. Kroker (1991), 'The hysterical male: one libido?', in A. Kroker and M. Kroker, *The Hysterical Male: New Feminist Fheory* (London: Macmillan), pp. x–xiv.

Landers, T. (1988), 'Bodies and anti-bodies: a crisis in representation', in C. Schneider and B. Wallis (eds), *Global Television* (New York: Wedge Press), pp. 281–298.

Lee, N. (2001), *Childhood and Society: Growing Up in an Age of Uncertainty* (Buckingham: Open University Press).

Lehman, P. (1993), *Running Scared: Masculinity and the Representation of the Male Body* (Philadelphia: Temple University Press).

Levine, J. (2002), *Harmful to Minors: The Perils of Protecting Children from Sex* (Minneapolis and London: University of Minnesota Press).

Lewis, J. and T. Knijn (2002), 'The politics of sex education policy in England and Wales and the Netherlands since the 1980s', *Journal of Social Policy*, 11:4, 669–694.

Lindsay, J., A. Smith and D. Rosenthal (1997), 'Secondary students, HIV/AIDS and sexual health', Monograph Series No. 3, Centre for the Studies of Sexually Transmissible Diseases, La Trobe University, Carlton.

Lupton, D. (1991), 'Apocalypse to banality: changes in metaphors about AIDS in the Australian press', *Australian Journal of Communication*, 18:2, 66–74.

Lupton, D. (1992), 'From complacency to panic: AIDS and heterosexuals in the Australian press, July 1986 to June 1988', *Health Education Research*, 7:1, 9–20.

Lupton, D. (1993), 'AIDS risk and heterosexuality in the Australian press', *Discourse and Society*, 4:3, 307–328.

Lupton, D. (1994), 'The condom in the age of AIDS: newly respectable or sill a dirty word? A discourse analysis', *Qualitative Health Research*, 4:3, 304–320.

Lupton, D. (1996), 'The feminine "AIDS body" in television drama', *Media International Australia*, 80 (May), 99–109.

Lupton, D., S. McCarthy and S. Chapman (1995), '"Panic bodies": discourses on risk and HIV antibody testing', *Sociology of Health and Illness*, 17:1, 89–109.

Lupton, D. and J. Tulloch (1996), '"Bringing home the reality of it": senior school students' responses to mass media portrayals of HIV/AIDS', *Australian Journal of Communication*, 23:1, 31–45.

Lupton, D. and J. Tulloch (1997), 'Senior school students' experiences and opinions of school based HIV-AIDS education', *Australian and*

New Zealand Journal of Public Health, 21:5, 531–538.
Lupton, D. and J. Tulloch (1998), 'The adolescent "unfinished body", reflexivity and HIV/AIDS risk', *Body & Society*, 4:2, 19–34.
Lury, C. (1998), *Prosthetic Culture* (London and New York: Routledge).
Lury, C. (2000), 'The united colors of diversity: essential and inessential culture', in S. Franklin, C. Lury and J. Stacey (eds), *Global Nature, Global Culture* (London and New Delhi: Sage), pp. 146–187.
MacKinnon, C. (1982), 'Feminism, marxism, method and the state: an agenda for theory', *Signs*, 7:3, 515–545.
MacKinnon, C. (1987a), 'Pleasure under patriarchy', in J. Geer and W. O'Donohue (eds), *Theories of Modern Sexuality* (New York: Plenham Press), pp. 65–90.
MacKinnon, C. (1987b), *Feminism Unmodified* (Cambridge, MA: Harvard University Press).
McClintock, A. (1992), 'Gonad the Barbarian and the Venus Flytrap: portraying the female and male orgasm', in L. Segal and M. McIntosh (eds), *Sex Exposed: Sexuality and the Pornography Debate* (London: Virago), pp. 111–131.
McGrath, R. (1990), 'Dangerous liaisons: health, disease and representation', in S. Gupta and T. Boffin (eds), *Ecstatic Antibodies: Resisting the AIDS mythology* (London: Rivers Oram Press, 1990).
Mills, J. (1992), 'Classroom conundrums: sex education and censorship', in L. Segal and M. McIntosh (ed.), *Sex Exposed: Sexuality and the Pornography Debate* (London: Virago), pp. 200–215.
Mitchell, K. and K. Wellings (2002), 'The role of ambiguity in sexual encounters between young people in England', *Culture, Health & Sexuality*, 4:4, 393–408.
Moore, S. M. and D. A. Rosenthal (1991), 'Condoms and coitus: adolescents' attitudes to AIDS and safe sex behaviour', *Journal of Adolescence*, 14, 211–227.
Moore, S. M. and D. Rosenthal (1992), 'The social context of adolescent sexuality: safe sex implications', *Journal of Adolescence*, 15, 415–435.
Moore, S. M. and D. Rosenthal (1993), *Sexuality and Adolescence* (London: Routledge).
Moran, J. P. (2000), *Teaching Sex: The Shaping of Adolescence in the 20th Century* (Cambridge, MA, and London: Harvard University Press).
Mort, F. (2000), *Dangerous Sexualities: Medico-moral Politics in England since 1830* (London and New York: Routledge, 2nd edition).
Mulvey, L. (1990), 'Visual pleasure and narrative cinema', in P. Erens (ed.), *Issues in Feminist Film Criticism* (Bloomington: Indiana University Press).
Munro, R. (1996), 'The consumption view of self: extension, exchange

and identity', in S. Edgell, K. Hethrington and A. Warde (eds), *Consumption Matters* (Cambridge: Blackwell).
Patton, C. (1986), 'Resistance and the erotic: reclaiming history, setting strategy as we face AIDS', *Radical America*, 20:6, 68–78.
Patton, C. (1989), 'Hegemony and orgasm – or the instability of heterosexual pornography', *Screen*, 30:12, 100–114.
Patton, C. (1990), *Inventing AIDS* (New York and London: Routledge).
Patton, C. (1991a), 'Visualising safe sex: when pedagogy and pornography collide', in D. Fuss (ed.), *Inside/Out* (New York and London: Routledge), pp. 373–386.
Patton, C. (1991b), 'Safe sex and the pornographic vernacular', in Bad Object Choices (ed.), *How Do I Look?* (Seattle: Bay Press).
Patton, C. (1993), '"With champagne and roses": women at risk from/in AIDS discourse', in C. Squire (ed.), *Women and AIDS, Psychological Perspectives* (London: Sage).
Patton, C. (1994), *Last Served? Gendering the HIV Pandemic* (London: Taylor and Francis).
Patton, C. (1995a), 'Between innocence and safety: epidemiologic and popular constructions of young people's need for safe sex', in J. Terry (ed.), *Deviant Bodies: Critical Perspectives on Difference in Science and Popular Culture* (Bloomington: Indiana University Press), pp. 338–357.
Patton, C. (1995b), 'Performativity and spatial distinction', in A. Parker and E. K. Sedgwick (eds), *Performativity and Performance* (London and New York: Routledge), pp. 173–196.
Patton, C. (1996), *Fatal Advice: How Safe Sex Education Went Wrong* (Durham and London: Duke University Press).
Patton, C. (1998), '"On me, not in me": locating affect in nationalism after AIDS', *Theory, Culture & Society*, 15:3–4, 355–373.
Pearce, S. (2004), 'Moulding the man: sex-education manuals for Australian boys in the 1950s', in C. Nelson and M. Martin (eds), *Sexual Pedagogies: Sex Education in Britain, Australia and America* (New York and England: Palgrave Macmillan).
Plummer, K. (1995), *Telling Sexual Stories* (London and New York: Routledge).
Poovey, M. (1998), 'Sex in America', *Critical Inquiry*, 224 (Winter), 366–392.
Porter, R. and L. Hall (1995), *The Facts of Life: The Creation of Sexual Knowledge in Britain, 1650–1950* (New Haven and London: Yale University Press).
Pringle, R. (1992), 'Absolute sex? Unpacking the sexuality/gender Relationship', in R. W. Connell and G. W. Dowsett (eds), *Rethinking Sex: Social Theory and Sexuality Research* (Melbourne: Melbourne University Press), pp. 76–101.

Richardson, D. (1990), 'AIDS education and women: sexual and reproductive issues', in P. Aggleton, P. Davies and G. Hart (eds), *AIDS: Individual, Cultural and Policy Dimensions* (Bristol: The Falmer Press), pp. 169–179.
Richardson, D. (1993), 'Sexuality and male dominance', in D. Richardon and V. Robinson (eds), *Introducing Women's Studies: Feminist Theory and Practice* (Basingstoke: Macmillan), pp. 74–98.
Richardson, D. (1994), 'AIDS: issues for feminism in the UK', in L. Doyal, J. Naidoo and T. Wilton (eds), *AIDS: Setting a Feminist Agenda* (London: Taylor and Francis), pp. 42–57.
Richardson, D. (1996), 'Contradictions in discourse: gender, sexuality and HIV/AIDS', in J. Holland and L. Adkins (eds), *Sex, Sensibility and the Gendered Body* (London: Macmillan).
Rigby, K., M. P. Brown, P. Anagnostou, M. W. Ross and B. Rosser (1989), 'Shock tactics to counter AIDS: the Australian experience', *Psychology and Health*, 3: 145–159.
Roberts, C., S. Kippax, M. Spongberg and J. Crawford (1996), '"Going down": oral sex, imaginary bodies and HIV', *Body & Society*, 2:3, 107–124.
Rosenthal, D. (1997), 'Understanding sexual coercion among young adolescents: communication clarity, pressure, and acceptance', *Archives of Sexual Behaviour*, 26:5, 481–493.
Rosenthal, D., S. Moore and I. Brumen (1990), 'Ethnic group differences in adolescents' responses to AIDS', *Australian Journal of Social Issues*, 25:3, 220–239.
Rosenthal, D., S. Moore and I. Flynn (1991),'Adolescent self-efficacy, self-esteem and sexual risk-taking', *Journal of Community & Applied Social Psychology*, 1: 77–88.
Rosenthal, D., A. Smith and R. de Visser (1997), 'Young people's condom use: an event specific analysis', *Venereology*, 10:2, 101–106.
Scott, S. (1987), 'Sex and danger: feminism and AIDS', *Trouble and Strife*, 11: 13–18.
Scott-Clark, C. and A. Levy (2005), 'Where it's really hurting', *The Guardian Weekend*, 10 September, 26–33.
Sedgwick, E. K. (1990), *Epistemology of the Closet* (New York and London: Harvester Wheatsheaf).
Segal, L. (1990), *Slow Motion: Changing Masculinities, Changing Men* (New Brunswick, NJ: Rutgers University Press).
Segal, L. (1992), 'Sweet sorrows, painful pleasures: pornography and the perils of heterosexual desire', in L. Segal and M. McIntosh (eds), *Sex Exposed: Sexuality and the Pornography Debate* (London: Virago), pp. 65–91.
Segal, L. (1994), *Straight Sex: The Politics of Pleasure* (London: Virago).

Segal, L. (1997), 'Feminist sexual politics and the heterosexual predicament', in L. Segal (ed.), *New Sexual Agendas* (London: Macmillan), pp. 77–89.
Segal, L. (1998), 'Only the literal: the contradictions of anti-pornography feminism', *Sexualities*, 1:1, 43–62.
Singer, L. (1993), *Erotic Welfare: Sexual Theory and Politics in the Age of Epidemic* (New York and London: Routledge).
Smart, C. (1996a), 'Collusion, collaboration and confession: on moving beyond the heterosexuality debate', in D. Richardson (ed.), *Theorising Heterosexuality: Telling It Straight* (Bristol: Open University Press), pp. 161–177.
Smart, C. (1996b), 'Desperately seeking post-heterosexual woman', in J. Holland and L. Adkins (eds), *Sex, Sensibility and the Gendered Body* (Basingstoke: Macmillan), pp. 222–241.
Smith, A. and D. Rosenthal (1997), 'Sex, alcohol and drugs? Young people's experience of Schoolies Week', *Australian and New Zealand Journal of Public Health*, 21:2, 175–180.
Snitow, A., C. Stansell and S. Thompson (1983), *Powers of Desire: The Politics of Sexuality* (New York: Monthly Review Press).
Sobo, E. J. (1995), *Choosing Unsafe Sex: AIDS-risk Denial Among Disadvantaged Women* (Philadelphia: University of Pennsylvania Press).
Speer, S. (2005), *Gender Talk: Feminism, Discourse and Conversation Analysis* (London and New York: Routledge).
Stanley, L. (1995), *Sex Surveyed* (London: Taylor and Francis).
Steinhardt, I. D. (1914), *Teen Sex Talks to Girls: 14 Years and Older* (Philadelphia: J. B. Lipincott Company).
Stephenson, N., S. Kippax and J. Crawford (2000), '"I couldn't imagine having sex with anyone else": young women's experience of trustworthiness in heterosexual relationships', in J. Ussher (ed.), *Women's Health: Contemporary International Perspectives* (London: Blackwell), pp. 105–114.
Stewart, F. (1991/92), 'Why it's not on to tell him: young women and safer sex', *Youth Issues Forum* (Summer), 6–7.
Stewart, F. (1994), 'Young women, safe sex and health promotion: why it's not on to tell him', *Australian Feminist Studies*, 20 (Summer), 25–34.
Stewart, F. (1999), '"Once you get a reputation, your life's like ... wrecked": the implications of reputation for young women's sexual health and well-being', *Women's Studies International Forum*, 22:3, 373–383.
Thomson, R. (1993), 'Unholy alliances: the recent politics of sex education', in J. Bristow and A. R. Wilson (eds), *Activating Theory: Lesbian,*

Gay and Bisexual Politics (London: Lawrence and Wishart), pp. 219–245.

Thomson, R. (1994), 'Moral rhetoric and public health pragmatism: the recent politics of sex education', *Feminist Review*, 48, 40–61.

Thomson, R. and J. Holland (1994), 'Young women and safer (hetero)sex: context, constraints and strategies', in S. Wilkinson and C. Kitzinger (eds), *Women and Health: Feminist Perspectives* (London: Taylor and Francis), pp. 13–33.

Thomson, R. and S. Blake (2002), 'Editorial', *Sex Education*, 2:3, 187–193.

Thorogood, N. (2000),'Sex education as disciplinary technique: policy and practice in England and Wales', *Sexualities*, 3:4, 425–438.

Treichler, P. (1987), 'AIDS, homophobia and biomedical discourse: an epidemic of signification', *Cultural Studies*, 1:3, 263–305.

Treichler, P. (1988), 'AIDS, gender and biomedical discourse: current contests for meaning', in E. Fee and D. M. Fox (eds), *AIDS: The Burdens of History* (Berkeley: University of California Press), pp. 190–266.

Treichler, P. (1992), 'Beyond Cosmo: AIDS, identity, and inscriptions of gender', *Camera Obscura*, 28, 21–76.

Tulloch, J. (1989), 'Australian television and the representation of AIDS', *Australian Journal of Communication*, 16 (December), 101–124.

Tulloch, J. (1992), 'Using TV in HIV/AIDS education: production and audience cultures', *Media Information Australia*, 5 (August), 10–27.

Tulloch, J. and D. Lupton (1997), *Television, AIDS and Risk: A Cultural Studies Approach to Health Education* (Sydney: Allen and Unwin).

Vance, C. (ed.) (1989), *Pleasure and Danger: Exploring Female Sexuality* (London and New York: Routledge).

Vance, C. (1994), 'Afterword: the war on culture continues 1989–94', in T. Gott (ed.), *Don't Leave Me This Way: Art in the Age of AIDS* (Melbourne, London and New York: Thames and Hudson), pp. 91–111.

Vasagar, J. and J. Borger (2005), 'Bush accused of AIDS damage to Africa', *The Guardian*, 30 August, pp. 1–2.

Waldby, C. (1995), 'Destruction: boundary erotics and refigurations of the heterosexual male body', in E. Probyn and E. Grosz (eds), *Sexy Bodies: The Strange Carnalities of Feminism* (London and New York: Routledge), pp. 266–277.

Waldby, C. (1996), *AIDS and the Body Politic: Biomedicine and Sexual Difference* (London and New York: Routledge).

Waldby, C., S. Kippax and J. Crawford (1990), 'Theory in the bedroom: a report from the Macquarie University AIDS Heterosexuality Project', *Australian Journal of Social Issues*, 25:3, 177–185.

Waldby, C., S. Kippax and J. Crawford (1991), 'Equality and eroticism: AIDS and the active/passive distinction', *Social Semiotics*, 1:2: 39–50.
Waldby, C., S. Kippax and J. Crawford (1993a), 'Research note: heterosexual men and "safe sex" practice', *Sociology of Health & Illness*, 15:2, 246–256.
Waldby, C., S. Kippax and J. Crawford (1993b), 'Cordon sanitaire: clean and unclean women in the AIDS discourse of young men', in P. Aggleton, P. Davies and G. Hart (eds), *AIDS: Facing the Second Decade* (London: The Falmer Press), pp. 29–39.
Warr, D. J. (2001), 'The importance of love and understanding: speculation on romance in safe sex health promotion', *Women's Studies International Forum*, 24:2, 241–252.
Watney, S. (1987), 'The spectacle of AIDS', *October*, 43 (Winter), 71–87.
Watney, S. (1988), 'Visual AIDS – advertising ignorance', in P. Aggleton and H. Homans (eds), *Social Aspects of AIDS* (London and Philadelphia: The Falmer Press), pp. 177–182.
Watney, S. (1989), *Policing Desire: Pornography, AIDS and the Media* (London: Metheun, 2nd edition).
Watney, S. (1991), 'School's out', in D. Fuss (ed.), *Inside/Out* (New York and London: Routledge), pp. 387–401.
Watney, S. (1992), 'Short-term companions: AIDS as popular entertainment', in A. Klusacek and K. Morrison (eds), *A Leap in the Dark: AIDS, Art and Contemporary Cultures* (Montreal: Vehicle Press), pp. 152–166.
Watney, S. (1994), *Practices of Freedom* (London: Rivers Oram Press).
Watson, J. (2003), 'Athlete's rape trial stirs controversy', 11Alive.com, 11 September, 1–3.
Weeks, J. (1981), *Sex, Politics and Society: The Regulation of Sexuality since 1800* (London: Longman).
Weeks, J. (1985), *Sexuality and Its Discontents* (London: Routledge and Kegan Paul).
Weeks, J. (1986), *Sexuality* (London: Ellis Horwood/Tavistock Publications).
Weeks, J. (1989), *Sex, Politics and Society: The Regulation of Sexuality since 1800* (London: Longman).
Weeks, J. (1991), *Against Nature: Essays on History, Sexuality and Identity* (London: Rivers Oram Press).
Weeks, J. (2000), *Making Sexual History* (London: Polity Press).
Weiss, G. (1999), *Body Images: Embodiment as Intercorporeality* (London and New York: Routledge).
Wellings, K., J. Field, A. Johnson and J. Wadsworth, *Sexual Behaviour in Britain: The National Survey of Sexual Attitudes and Lifestyles* (London: Penguin).

Widdicombe, S. and R. Woofit (1995), *The Language of Youth Subculture* (Brighton: Harvester).
Wight, D. (1993a), 'Constraint or cognition? Young men and safer heterosexual sex', in P. Aggleton, P. Davies and G. Hart (eds), *AIDS: Facing the Second Decade* (London: The Falmer Press), pp. 41–60.
Wight, D. (1993b), 'A re-assessment of health education on HIV/AIDS for young heterosexuals', *Health Education Research*, 8:4, 473–483.
Wight, D. (1994a), 'Assimilating safer sex: young heterosexual men's understanding of "safer sex"', in P. Aggleton, P. Davies and G. Hart (eds), *AIDS: Foundations for the Future* (London: Taylor and Francis), pp. 97–109.
Wight, D. (1994b), 'Boys' thoughts and talk about sex in a working class locality in Glasgow', *Sociological Review*, 42:4, 703–738.
Wight, D. (1996), 'Beyond the predatory male: the diversity of young men's discourses to describe heterosexual relationships', in L. Adkins and V. Merchant (eds), *Sexualising the Social* (Basingstoke: Macmillan), pp. 145–172.
Wight, D. (1999), 'Cultural factors in young heterosexual men's perception of HIV risk', *Sociology of Health and Illness*, 21:6, 735–758.
Williams, L. (1990), *Hard Core: Power, Pleasure and the 'Frenzy of the Visible'* (London: Pandora).
Williamson, J. (1989), 'Every virus tells a story: the meaning of HIV and AIDS', in E. Carter and S. Watney (eds), *Taking Liberties* (London: Serpent's Tail), pp. 69–80.
Wilton, T. (1994), 'Feminism and the erotics of health promotion', in L. Doyal, J. Naidoo and T. Wilton (eds), *AIDS. Setting a Feminist Agenda* (London: Taylor and Francis), pp. 80–95.
Wilton, T. (1996), *Finger-Licking Good* (London: Cassell, 1996).
Wilton, T. (1997), *EnGendering AIDS* (London: Sage).
Wilton, T. and P. Aggleton (1991), 'Condoms, coercion and control: heterosexuality and the limits to HIV/AIDS education', in P. Aggleton, G. Hart and P. Davies (eds), *AIDS: Responses, Interventions and Care* (London: The Falmer Press), pp. 149–156.
Wolpe, A. (1987), 'Sex in schools: back to the future', *Feminist Review*, 27 (September), 37–47.
Wood, N. (1985), 'Foucault on the history of sexuality: an introduction', in V. Beechey and J. Donald (eds), *Subjectivity and Social Relations* (Milton Keynes: Open University Press), pp. 156–175.
Wyatt-Seal, D. and A. A. Ehrhardt (1999), 'Heterosexual men's attitudes toward the female condom', *AIDS Education and Prevention*, 11:2, 93–106.
Wyn, J. (1994), 'Young women and sexually transmitted diseases: the

issues for public health', *Australian Journal of Public Health*, 18:1 (1994), 32–39.
Younge, G. (2004), 'Deep South divided by rape case', *The Guardian*, 23 January, 17.

Index

abstinence education 17, 25, 27, 30, 121
ACT UP 65
Adkins, L. 75
adolescence
  AIDS 5, 7, 11, 137
  class and 29–31, 67
  ethnicity and 72–3, 76
  futurity and 27–30, 31, 33, 35, 67, 71, 73–5, 136–9
  race and 29–31, 66–7, 118–20
  safer sex discourse and 121–3, 129
  sexual regulation and 33, 136, 139
  the unfinished body and 32, 35, 52–4
'African AIDS' 5, 25
African Americans
  condoms and 118–20
  the media and 65–7
  youth and 67
AIDS media representations
  the condom 58, 60–5, 67, 70–3, 76
  de-gaying AIDS and 60
  heteronormativity and 68
  heterosexuality and 57–61, 67–72
  homophobia and 6, 8–10, 16, 46
  homosexuality and 58–61, 69–70
  public health campaigns and 57–73, 77
  racism and 65–6
  whiteness and 73, 77
Altman, D. 56
Ang, I. 72

'barebacking' 9
Bashford, A. 15–16
Berlant, L. 68–9
Berridge, V. 58–60
Bersani, L. 6, 10–11

Bland, L. 18, 98
Bordo, S. 80, 83–4, 87
Brandt, A. 7, 63–4
Bravmann, S. 2–4
Brown, W. 82
Browne, J. and Minichiello, V. 96, 100, 130–3
Buston, K. and Wight, D. 34–5
Butler, J. 93, 105, 120–1, 129

Carter, J. 14–15
Chapman, S. and Hodgson, J. 129–30
children
  the child 27–8, 70
  childhood and 35
  sexuality and 7, 26–7
christian right 25–6, 120
class 3, 6, 11, 14, 17, 20, 29–31, 37, 40–1, 51, 65, 67, 69, 72–5, 119, 138
clause 28 21, 60, 88
Cohen, C. 65–6
condoms
  the classroom 25–6, 29, 32–5, 121
  consent and 119–22, 124, 127–8
  queer sexualities and 3–4, 91–4
  reflexivity and 74–7
  sex research and 40, 45, 51–2, 104–6, 111–12, 114–16, 121, 125–34
  sexual stories and 49, 50, 71, 119–21, 127, 129, 132
condom use
  female empowerment and 100, 124, 126
  as feminising 96–7, 99–101, 129, 132
  sexual negotiation and 39, 102, 117,

131–2, 138
Connell, R. W. 112
consent 12, 21, 35, 39, 116–17, 119–22, 124, 127–9, 131, 133–5
Conway, M. 79, 93–4
Coward, R. 89, 99
Crawford, J., Kippax, S. and Waldby, C. 101
Cronin, A. 67–8

Dean, T. 9
D'Emilio, J. and Freedman, E. 24
Dixon v. The State 118–21
Dowsett, G. 46–7
Durham, M. 20
Dworkin, A. 81
Dyer, R. 86

Edelman, L. 86
empowerment 124, 126
ethnicity 75–6, 138
Ericksen, J. 36–41

female condom 114
Ferguson, R. 67
Findlay, H. 91–2
Flood, M. 121
Flowers, P. 9
Foucault, M. 32–3, 53, 98, 103
Franklin, S., Lury, C. and Stacey, J. 73
Fraser, M. 49–50
Fung, R. 85
Fuqua, J. 60
Fuss, D. 68

Gagnon, J. and Simon, W. 37–8
Gamson, J. 2–5, 64
Gavey, N. 112, 126, 131
gay men
  HIV 8–10, 48, 60
  the media and 6–7, 10, 11
  safer sex and 3–4, 8, 79
  sex research and 40, 43, 45, 47
gender
  heterosexuality 39, 82–3, 104, 124, 126, 129, 134
  identity and 11–12, 84–5
  media representations and 63, 78, 81, 90
  performativity and 83, 97, 105, 112, 137
  safer sex discourse and 77, 122, 126–8
  social constructionism and 122–3, 128
Gilman, S. 7, 61–2
Gordon, A. 54, 138
Gott, T. 60
Griffin, G. 93
Griffin, K. 126–7
'Grim Reaper' 57–8, 61–2, 64, 67, 72, 77, 121
Grosz, E. 80, 107–8, 113, 115

Hage, G. 77
Halberstam, J. 84
Hall, L. 14, 17, 19
Hall, S. 13–14
Hammonds, E. 65–6
Hampshire, J. 18–19
Haraway, D. 117
Harre, R. 50
heteronormativity 47, 72, 79, 93
Hillier, L. et al. 130–1
HIV treatments 9
Holland et al. 51, 100–2, 104–5, 111–12, 123–5, 128, 131,134
Hollway, W. 97, 102–3

'Iceberg' advertisement 59
identity
  gender 11–12, 75, 77–9, 84–5, 87, 95, 97, 101, 107, 112, 128, 136
  national and 12, 57, 69, 77
  self and 68, 87, 109–11, 115–17
  sexual and 7, 11, 12, 20, 22–3, 36, 41–2, 49, 50, 60, 68, 71, 76–7, 79, 81, 85, 87–8, 90–4, 114
'If it's not on, it's not on' 97, 100, 104, 106, 120
Irvine, J. 26–8, 120–1

Jackson, S. 19–20
Jackson, S. and Scott, S. 102–3
Jagose, A. 94
Jeffreys, S. 81, 93–4
Juffer, J. 79, 90–1
Juhasz, A. 61–2

Kaite, B. 78, 89
Kappeler, S. 81
Kimmel, M. 99
Kinsey, A. 37
Kipnis, L. 91
Kippax, S. and Kinder, P. 45–6

Kroker, A. and Kroker, M. 80

Landers, T. 60
Lee, N. 35, 117
Lehman, P. 86
lesbians
  AIDS discourse 47, 60, 94
  AIDS research and 40, 42–5, 50
  safer sex and 92–4
Levine, J. 27
Lewis, J. and Knijn, T. 22–3
Lindsay, J., Smith, A. and Rosenthal, D. 51–2, 105
Lupton, D. 57–8, 61, 68
Lupton, D. and Tulloch, J. 32–3, 52–3, 57, 68, 70–1
Lury, C. 76, 116

McClintock, A. 80, 86
McGrath, R. 61, 63
MacKinnon, C. 81–2
masculinity
  the male body 78–80, 83, 86–7, 91, 93, 96–9, 103–4, 108–13, 124
  the male sex drive and 39, 97–8, 100–5
  safer sex and 80–1, 87, 96–7, 99–105, 113–17, 123, 131, 137
  without men 84, 93
Mills, J. 20
Mitchell, K. and Wellingsm K. 134
Moore, S. and Rosenthal, D. 73–6, 124–5, 133
moral panic theory 6–7
Moran, J. 13–14, 24–5, 29
Mort, F. 7, 16–18
Mulvey, L. 85
Munro, R. 17

Patton, C. 29–31, 66–7, 70, 79–80, 85, 87, 102, 122
Pearce, S. 17
penis
  AIDS 80–1, 86
  heterosex and 111–13, 124
  porn and 82–6
phallus
  its deconstruction and 82–4, 87, 92–4
  the lesbian and 92–3
  phallocentricism and 1, 80–1, 84, 87, 93–4, 137
  pornography and 80, 82–4, 86, 92

Plummer, K. 47–8
Poovey, M. 42–3, 50
pornography
  AIDS 78–9, 92
  the come shot and 85–6
  feminist debates and 79, 81–93
  gay porn and 79, 91
  the gaze and 84–5, 89
  lesbian porn and 79, 92–4
  its production and 84
  safer sex and 87–8, 91–4
  sexual difference and 86, 89, 95
  women consumers and 90
Porter, R. and Hall, L. 5
power
  disciplinary 1–2, 11, 13, 22, 27, 33, 53, 121, 136, 139
  male and 81–3, 87, 102, 104, 111, 122–7
Pringle, R. 103

racism 29, 30, 65–7, 72–3, 75–6, 118–19, 141
rape 118–20
regulation
  adolescent sexuality 5, 7, 11, 13, 15, 22–3, 28, 136–7, 139
  AIDS and sexuality 1–2, 7, 27, 88, 136
  women's sexuality and 62–3
repressive hypothesis 103
research methods
  qualitative methods 43–8, 50, 52–4, 71
  quantitative methods and 42–3, 46, 52, 70–1
Richardson, D. 99–100, 107, 114, 122–3, 133
Rosenthal, D. et al. 73, 75–6, 105–6

safer sex education
  in magazines 64–5
  SHARE package 34–5
  targeting approach 23, 27–30, 67
  on television 56–61, 64–6, 69–70
safer sex practice
  negotiation and 34, 39, 102, 117, 126–7, 131–3, 138
  pleasure and 99–101, 104–5, 125–7
  power and 100–2, 122–3, 126, 134
school sex education policies
  Australia 31–3, 52–3
  Britain 18–23

North America 14, 23–30
Scotland 34–5
Scott, S. 99
Sedgwick, E. K. 27
Segal, L. 80–3, 86–7, 96, 110, 112
sex education
  boys 13, 17, 35
  class and 14, 17, 29
  the future and 16, 20, 23, 27, 29–30, 33, 35
  girls and 18, 21, 34
  the nation and 14–15
  public health and 15–16
  purity organisations and 17
  race and 14, 16–17, 29, 30
  sexuality and 15–17, 24
  the social hygiene movement and 17
Sex in America (survey) 41–2
sexology 98
sex research
  adolescence 37–40, 49–54, 70–3, 121, 125, 127, 129–35
  gay standpoint and 45–6
  heteronormativity and 41–5, 47, 52, 54
  methods and 41–2, 45
  social researchers and 37, 41, 44, 46, 48, 52–3, 71–6, 120, 123–4
Sexual Attitudes and Lifestyles (survey) 43–4
sexual behaviour
  first heterosex 101, 111–12, 129, 132
  safer sex and 101, 121–2, 128–34
  unsafe sex and 96–7, 99–102, 123–4, 127–8
sexual difference 108–10, 113, 115
  the condom 113–16
  porn and 86, 89, 95
sexual diseases
  plague imagery 7–8
  syphilis and 14, 62
  veneral disease and 63
sexual epidemic 1, 62
sexual knowledge 5, 7, 27
sexual speech 26–7, 120
sexual stories
  adolescence 49–50
  AIDS and 47–8
  safer sex and 47–9
sex survey
  adolescence 37–9, 51–2
  heterosexuality and 41–2, 44–5

homosexuality and 40–5
lesbians and 40, 42–4
Singer, L. 1, 61–2, 80
Smart, C. 110
Smith, A. and Rosenthal, D. 106
Sobo, E. J. 66
Speer, S. 126, 135
Stanley, L. 43–5
Stephenson, N. *et al.* 109
Stewart, F. 127

Thomson, R. 20–3, 51, 100
Thorogood, N. 22
'Tombstone' advertisement 59, 64
Treichler, P. 60–2, 64–5
Tulloch, J. 57, 61, 70–1
Tulloch, J. and Lupton, D. 58, 72–3

unsafe sex
  adolescents 23, 50–2, 77, 96, 97, 99–102, 105, 123–4, 127–8
  gay men and 9
  heterosexual men and 96–7, 102–4, 123–4, 138

Vance, C. 60

Waldby, C. 80, 83, 87, 99–100, 104, 106, 108–10, 114–15
Waldby, C., Kippax, S. and Crawford, J. 106, 110, 115–16
Warr, D. 134
Watney, S. 6–8, 60–1, 87–8
Weeks, J. 19–21, 58, 98
Weiss, G. 112–13
Wellcome Trust 43
whiteness 15–16, 30–1, 65, 67, 69–70, 72–3, 77, 119, 138
Wight, D. 57, 73–4, 129–30, 132
Williams, L. 80, 84
Williamson, J. 60–1
Wilton, T. 80, 87, 89, 101, 107, 114, 123–4
Wilton, T. and Aggleton, P. 100, 122–4
Wolpe, A. 19–20
women's bodies
  AIDS representations 62
  health education and 96, 106–7
  safer sex and 100, 107–9, 115–16
Wood, N. 98
Wyn, J. 127

Lightning Source UK Ltd.
Milton Keynes UK
UKOW030247270313

208232UK00008B/212/P